"In her book, *The End of Living Large*, Sue Speake gives readers an honest look at her quest for weight loss and how she came to terms with her unhealthy relationship to food. Sue tells a story that many who have struggled with their weight will relate to, as she gives readers a detailed account of what supported her and what sabotaged her along the way. Unlike many others Sue's story ends well and she offers readers hope, giving them specific tips in her desire that others can improve their own relationship with eating and weight."

—CAROLYN COSTIN ,M.A., M.ED., MFT, FAED, Chief Clinical Officer, Monte Nido & Affiliates

The End of Living Large is filled with valuable advice for anybody seeking to achieve good health. It illustrates an innovative, progressive plan that is designed to normalize weight that is sustainable and lasting. It is a must read for all of us motivated to succeed in our quest for healthy living."

—ALCIRA SAHAMI, MD, Child, Adolescent, and Adult Psychiatrist

"This is an easy, readable, and at times fun approach to changing the way we eat. Sue's use of HRRTs is a clever approach for those who struggle with weight loss, making it more obtainable. Utilizing her MicroSteps® philosophy is brilliant for those who know that we have to do it one-step at a time. The combination of practical ideas, good recipes, and common sense make this an important read for anyone wanting to get a handle on their weight loss."

—KATE QUINN TANDY, Ph.D.

"In today's fast-paced world, we often try to change our eating patterns equally fast in order to lose weight. However, as quick as change comes, it can also leave us. Ms. Speake's book offers a shift in this perspective of fleeting weight loss by providing instead a view of health and non-diet eating that leads to permanent weight loss and a kinder, more fulfilling sense of ourselves."

—MICHELYN DEVINE, Psy.D.

"How refreshing to read a "diet" book that has nothing to do with dieting. Sue lets the world in on her weight loss secret—DON'T DIET. This book is so easy to read and follow. Sue's journey through her own weight loss is real and full of tons of practical advice and insight. As a therapist who works with clients who have issues with obesity as well as traditional eating disorders, I believe Sue's ideas can work for all."

—**MICHELE PARMLEY,** Licensed Clinical Social Worker

The End of Living LARGE

The End of Living LARGE

Weight Loss in MicroSteps®
When You Have a Lot to Lose

Sue Speake, LMFT

SPEAKE PRESS
BAKERSFIELD, CA

For more information contact:
Speake Press
P.O. Box 22254
Bakersfield, CA 93390

Paperback: 978-0-9864418-0-6
eBook: 978-0-9864418-1-3

Library of Congress Control Number: 2015901019

DISCLAIMER: The information in this book is not intended as diagnostic for mental or physical health issues, a substitute for consultation with medical professionals, or replacement for treatment by a licensed mental health professional. You should consult a physician in matters relating your health and particularly in respect to any symptoms that may require diagnosis or medical attention. You should consult a licensed mental health professional for mental health evaluations and concerns.

Book Design by Dotti Albertine

To my mother,
who taught me how to
cook Texas style,
sew a dress from a pattern,
and never give up.

Contents

PART ONE

The End of Living Large

CHAPTER 1

Living Large

AT THE AGE OF FIFTY, I gave up dieting forever and decided just to be fat. For about six years, I ignored weight gain, struggled with the challenges of living in an obese body, ate everything I wanted, and almost believed I did not care. All the while, I felt horrified about how I looked. I could have won an Oscar for how well I faked confidently walking into business meetings and events, while feeling humiliated to the core about my appearance. By age fifty-five, I weighed three hundred and fifteen pounds. I was working the most stressful job of my life and looking the worst I had ever looked. I tried to convince myself that it was who I was on the inside that mattered.

My behaviors told another story. I avoided anyone who had not seen me since I was an average size. I remember running into an old friend, an artist who happens to sculpt human figures. When she saw me, she reached up and gently touched my cheeks that had gotten much fatter. She looked at me with compassion and removed her hand. I thought, "She knows my shame." I felt so incongruent; my intelligence, professional expertise, sophistication, people skills, nothing matched the obese person others were seeing. I knew I was much more stylish inside than anyone would have ever guessed. It was difficult to be obese and work as a psychotherapist where colleagues not only dressed professionally but also could often identify many issues just looking at you.

Never being a person to jump onto the latest diet bandwagon, the only diet I'd ever used was counting calories. I counted calories from ages 28 to 50. I wrote down every bite I took and the calorie counts for twenty plus years! I lost and regained weight a few times during those years. At first, I counted calories alone.

A few years later, while trying the buddy system with a psychologist friend, I ended up gaining weight. We held each other accountable, talked daily about what we ate, counted calories and fiber, as well as weighed and measured each other. While I loved being in the process with my friend and having the support, it backfired on me. I ended up larger than when we started, most likely because my inner adolescent rebels against having to report to someone or be held accountable for what I eat. After years of calorie counting, I quit. I could not diet any more.

Why did I give up dieting? I became discouraged. I knew I could lose weight but I was tired of counting calories, feeling deprived, and doing without the foods I liked and wanted. I got tired of people telling me what to eat, how to eat it, and when to eat. I did not want to talk about emotional eating or using food to solve problems; I wanted to live my life like the people who do not seem to have weight problems. It was just too frustrating to go through the guilty feelings every time I ate pizza or ice cream. I felt I could no longer live my life in guilt, controlled by food; so, I quit dieting and ate whatever I wanted.

In the beginning of the post calorie counting *no diet years*, my eating was out of control. I was like a teenager with a new driver's license who volunteers to do all the family errands, drives too fast, happily picks up younger siblings from school, and offers to go to the store for Mom. Once the newness wears off, most drivers settle down, drive when they need to go somewhere, and generally in a responsible manner. Of course, some never settle down and still drive too fast but you get the idea. At first, I was eating fast food daily, enjoying cakes, sweets, chips, and plenty of pizza. I was binging on everything I had denied myself over those long years of counting calories. I was eating whatever happened to be the quickest, easiest, and tastiest. I was completely self indulgent, although, it took a while before I could do it without guilt. Getting to the point where I could eat badly *without guilt* was actually part of the healing process. I needed to recover from the trauma of all those years of deprivation and calorie counting. At the time, I thought this was my new way of life and I would remain obese forever. I had completely given up.

The giving up was about more than just what I was eating. I stopped wearing fashionable clothes. I wore clothes that were extra large, baggy, and did not fit. I purchased clothes that were of poorer quality than the clothes of my thinner days and had only one pair of shoes that I wore daily. I quit wearing jewelry and accessories. I had stopped trying to look good in a fashionable world. While I always kept myself clean, did my hair, and wore make-up, I told myself that I only needed to blend in and be comfortable.

Unfortunately, I was not blending in at all but did not realize it at the time. I had moved to a small town and thought that no one knew who I really was and it did not matter. The thing is that for most of my adult life I had dressed fashionably and cared about how I presented myself publicly. This radical change could have easily led to depression, if I had not been so successful in my professional life.

How Did I Get to This Place?

Like many young women, I always felt fat and measured myself against an unattainable standard of *perfect*. It was only in looking back at old photographs of myself did I realize that I actually had been an average size until I hit my late thirties. I wore sizes 8 to 12 until I was around age forty. After that, my weight increased slowly until I became a full-time therapist and then I gained quickly.

It's hard to pinpoint exactly why I gained so much weight. There were the normal life stressors including financial problems, successes, failures, and the career change from teaching to adjusting to being a full-time therapist. Of course, a teacher is physically moving all the time while a therapist mostly sits and listens or talks all day. As a therapist, I got off work late in the evening, grabbed fast food on the way home, and then went to bed—a recipe for weight gain, a Habit that was not serving my health. (I'll discuss "Habits" later.)

From ages forty to fifty, my weight increased from 200 pounds to 292 pounds. This happened in spite of the fact that those were happy years, with a good social life, and family support. At the age of fifty, weighing 292 pounds, I gave up my private practice in Burbank, California, a city in Los Angeles County. I relocated to the smaller town of Bakersfield, California and accepted, what turned out to be, a very stressful position with a county mental health department. When I stepped into the new job, I stepped into a different culture. In the Los Angeles area, people were weight conscious and there would never have been the daily doughnuts in the work place but this was common in the new location, where there were the doughnuts along with sodas with sugar, and multiple potlucks with tasty but unhealthy foods. I could not resist and started to gain weight almost immediately due to the job stress and the food temptations all around me. It was at this point that I gave up and began to eat whatever I wanted, determined never to go on another diet.

Ironically, this is where my healing from the trauma of living large began. Initially, *giving up* felt like freedom. I had a sense of relief. It actually took a couple of years of being completely out of control before things started to change. Did I continue to gain weight for a while? You bet I did. I eventually hit 315 pounds. I'd heard for years that if you put healthy choices in front of children and leave them alone they eventually eat a balanced diet. I don't know if this is true but in my own case, I eventually got so tired of the way I felt after eating sweets and fast food that I began to seek out healthier foods and started cooking for myself.

A New Kind of Freedom

As it turns out, *giving up* and eating whatever I wanted was the smartest thing I ever did. I don't recommend it as a rule but it allowed me to heal from the trauma of dieting all those years. In 2009, I found myself beginning to do less *acting out* with food. That is to say, I was eating less junk food and had fewer moments of binge eating. I began to be able to say no to myself and to make healthier choices. This was a new kind of freedom; one that I had never experienced before. I was eating what I wanted to eat and yet making healthier choices, although in the beginning I must say that the healthier choices had a lot to do with wanting to avoid the discomfort of feeling overly full and bloated.

Being a psychotherapist, I decided to self-observe so that I could figure out what had happened to cause the healthier eating and changes in Habits. It happened so slowly that it is almost impossible to describe. I noticed that eventually I was able to say no to fast food or pizza without feeling deprived or left out. I knew I could have pizza or fast food any time I wanted it, so I would make a healthier choice because it was easier to live with myself after the eating was over. I began to look for foods that made me feel good after I ate them. I noticed that sweets and caffeine late at night caused me to lose sleep, interfering with my work. I also noticed that my joints swelled after the fast food; I think it might have been the sodium. I would choose something healthier and tell myself not to worry; I could have the cheeseburger and fries tomorrow. Somehow, the tomorrows got further and further apart and I was eating healthier and still eating everything I wanted to eat. My *wants* were changing.

At this point, I begin to explore ways to continue changing my lifestyle so that I could regain my pride, self-esteem, physical health, and feel better about myself in general. I admitted to myself that how we present ourselves to others does matter and has a powerful impact on our lives either in a positive or negative manner. I began to look for ways to continue in this move forward that I had stumbled upon quite accidentally.

"Just Change Your Lifestyle"

Most diets result in weight loss, but then you're told you need to "change your lifestyle to maintain the weight loss." What they fail to tell you is *how* to change your lifestyle. "By eating healthy and exercising," they say. Of course, but what does that have to do with changing one's lifestyle? What is *lifestyle* anyway? How does one change a lifestyle when the average person cannot even clearly define the term? Most people think it just means eat right, exercise, find no comfort in food, eat stuff you don't really like, and go to the gym. We do not have the slightest clue as to *how* to change our lifestyle permanently to support the weight loss. Therefore, we regain the weight, go on another diet, lose weight again, and then gain it back plus more. Meanwhile, the diet industry is making millions!

About The End of Living Large

This book is going to provide insight into what is involved in changing your *lifestyle* and offer ideas as to how to make those lifestyle changes stick. I define lifestyle as "a way of life or style of living that reflects the attitudes and values of a person or group." I'll share with you how I developed a way of life or style of living that allows me to completely be myself, eat what I want, and remain a healthy person in an average size body. My *wants* simply changed; at least that is what happened to me. My hope is that you will find the same for yourself.

When a lifestyle is changed, exciting and surprising things happen. It may look like a diet to others but we have a secret— *this is not a diet!* You are eating whatever you want to eat. Your *wants* have simply changed. You gain pleasure from foods to which, in the past, you felt indifferent. You do not find yourself missing anything or feeling deprived. You feel satisfied. When you do eat something that everyone else says is off limits for a healthy diet, you just enjoy it and move on. You notice that somehow, you are no longer overeating and you wonder when and how that happened.

Surprise! It happened! You have arrived. The guilt and shame are gone. The long journey is over; you can now live your life in peace free from weight issues. After all, you have changed your *lifestyle* so all you have left to do is to live your life in style and with pride.

Habits, Routines, Rituals and Traditions—HRRTs

People are creatures of Habits, Routines, Rituals, and Traditions (HRRTs). I mentioned one of these, Habits, earlier. We gain comfort from our HRRTs and turn to them as a way of reducing the feelings of upset or anxiety. Most weight loss programs/diets *"flood"* people with changes that they are unable to maintain. This *"flooding"* creates anxiety. While the anxiety is generally subconscious and not of great significance in the beginning, the anxiety eventually increases and causes a return to old Habits, Routines, Rituals, and Traditions for comfort. When people eat less food than their body needs, they lose weight. While most diet plans result in people losing weight, going on a diet does not necessarily mean a person will end up healthy. In fact, the opposite is often true. People return to Habits, Routines, Rituals, and Traditions during celebrations, as well as during times of stress and crisis. They provide a comfort zone that pulls us back to our old ways of eating and behaving.

Not all comfort zones are equal; some are healthy and support healthy living. Some are unhealthy and only contribute to unhealthy living and an unhealthy body. Habits, Routines, Rituals, and Traditions are comfort zones that change over time as we age, mature, enter different life situations, marry, divorce, have children, relocate our home, change schools, make new friends, or change jobs.

While the focus of this book is about managing over-weight issues, the principles apply to any weight management issues, including the need to gain weight. There is no diet plan; instead, you will achieve a *lifestyle change* by addressing the Habits, Routines, Rituals, and Traditions that are preventing you freedom from the shame, trauma, and the emotional pain of unsuccessful weight management.

Becoming aware of dysfunctional Habits, Routines, Rituals, and Traditions and slowly implementing healthier HRRTs is not easy and is not a quick fix, but it can be a permanent resolution to keeping the weight off and living a healthier life. Remember, your body did not become unhealthy overnight and it will not return to a healthier state in a couple of months. It takes time to change a lifestyle. The body becomes unhealthy due to dysfunctional comfort zones or HRRTs; it only makes sense that developing healthy ones will have a positive impact on one's body. This is why I believe that one must first change the lifestyle and the *healthy, average size body* will follow. The majority of our HRRTs are automatic, assumed, or mindless. Intentionally establishing healthy ones help prevent you from automatically returning to unhealthy comfort foods. As your HRRTs become intentional, you develop the power to control your weight forever. You have options and choices that remove you from being a victim of the emotional and physical trauma of yo-yo dieting.

The Magic of MicroSteps®

How does one change Habits, Routines, Rituals, and Traditions? Below, I'll introduce you to the concept of MicroSteps, a simple approach that provided me with the willpower to make permanent changes that are helping me maintain a healthy, average size body.

By making changes very slowly, over time, and in MicroSteps, we can find the same comfort in healthier Habits, Routines, Rituals, and Traditions—*new* HRRTs, you could say. Will this change our wants and our eating forever? Will we ever be able to experience an apple as comfort food? If we avoid the dieting that *floods* and creates anxiety, will this help us avoid regaining the weight?

I believe so and this is where I started my journey. I am finding comfort in new ways of eating, supported by healthier new HRRTs, and do not need to diet to lose weight. I am losing weight slowly without dieting.

I remember when the idea of making changes in my eating felt threatening and caused me to feel anxious. When it's been a long week, and you're looking forward to the every Friday night dinner of ribs and fries at your favorite restaurant, the thought of change can create a feeling of panic. This is where MicroSteps play such an important role.

Years ago, I had a patient who wanted to go to a 12 Step Alcoholics Anonymous Meeting but was too anxious to walk into the meeting. We discussed it; the patient agreed to spend the first few weeks just driving by the meeting but not stopping the car. Next, the patient drove past the meeting and slowed down the car. The next step was to stop and park the car without getting out. Finally, the patient was able to sit in the car and watch people come and go to the meeting. Eventually, the patient parked the car a little closer to the meeting. Finally, the patient went into the meeting; the last I heard this brave soul had 10 plus years clean and sober. He'd become active in the program, attending different meetings, and sharing his story in front of the groups.

It's all about MicroSteps. When we push ourselves too hard and too abruptly, we trigger a flight or fight response and the battle is lost because we return to old familiar negative HRRTs, our comfort zone.

What's Next?

So, that is where this book is going. You will be introduced to the positive and negative influence of Habits, Routines, Rituals, and Traditions (HRRTs) on weight management, and learn how to substitute some *new* HRRTs. We will discuss the impact of abruptly dieting and the resulting anxiety that leads one back to unhealthy eating and comfort foods. Learning to look at the process of achieving a healthy, average size body by means of MicroSteps will bring it all together.

So, relax and take your time. The process is slow, read slowly, make changes slowly, and celebrate every little thing you accomplish. For example, you have read chapter one. That means you are closer to getting a healthy, average size body. Do not be surprised if you end up eating in similar ways occasionally as some of the folks who are still dieting. Just because you want to eat an apple instead of a bag of French fries, does not mean you are on a diet.

You do not need to run out and buy healthy foods. There is no need for a calorie counter and I would encourage you to eat tomorrow as you ate today. Relax, the answers are inside you; the information provided as you continue reading will help you reach deeply inside and find your way. All you need to do to begin the journey to a healthy, average size body is to relax and resolve the following.

Resolve

- To end all diets

- To expect no quick fixes as you take MicroSteps

- To eat whatever you want

- To gain and seek knowledge

- To self-observe your Habits, Routines, Rituals, and Traditions so that you become aware of what, when, where, and why you eat

- To understand the impact of others on your life and weight management

- To patiently allow your body to adjust slowly, over time, in MicroSteps, until it becomes a healthy, average size

- To change your *wants*, by slowly substituting *new* HRRTs, so that you may become an healthy, average size without dieting; while at the same time, being comfortable with what you are eating, what you are wearing, how you are moving, and with your life

❧ ❧ ❧

Today, eat whatever you want.

Trust your wants to change one *MicroStep* at a time.

Remember, it was the turtle who won the race!

Chapter 2

The First MicroSteps®

It's not where you start it's where you finish. Say you could go anywhere in the world, so you decide to visit New York City. You create a travel plan and end up in New York. While you might take one route, somebody else might take another, and a third person yet another. One person might choose to start the trip immediately, another would have to save up the money, another might want to deal with a fear of flying, or another could want to resolve a family situation before starting the journey. However, everyone who really wanted to get to New York City could get there.

Did you ever hear the expression *"first things first?"* To begin this process you must prepare, pack for the trip, and make sure you have what you need for the journey. As you read this chapter, do not be discouraged if you need to do a little preparation. Taking the time to identify a good starting place for your unique situation will help you succeed along the way.

If you've decided that being a *healthy, average size* is your goal, then simply begin your journey. Once you decide where to start, the rest of the journey will become obvious. This may sound a little vague but it will become clear as we continue. The exciting thing is that you can always identify a new starting place. There is no failure in this journey. Since there is no such thing as perfection, if you miss an issue, never fear, you will deal with it as it comes up. Have you ever gotten lost on the way to a destination? Did you ever have to stop and get directions or turn around and try a different route? Do not expect perfection; it does not exist! Believe me, that is good news.

The journey may feel bumpy at first and you may stumble, however, if you continue to put one foot in front of the other, you will find your way.

Things That Helped in the Beginning

Several experiences helped me as I slowly became open to managing my weight issue. I want to share some of these things with you. My hope is that they will inspire and help you decide what will be your starting place.

Under the Radar

I did not tell anyone what I was doing until I had lost almost fifty pounds and people started noticing my weight loss and mentioning it. Doing it *under the radar* helped because I tend to rebel against diet advice and did not want to act out with eating just because yet another thin person wanted to tell me how to lose weight. When an obese person starts a diet, people not only give you a lot of advice but they also expect you to fail. They may not say it directly, but you can tell by their facial expressions, and by what they do say. You know, the artificial "good for you" response when you say, "I have lost five pounds." When someone asked me how I was losing the weight, I just said, "I am eating healthy." I played it down and did not share my secret. All along, I was writing this book about how to lose weight and keep it off.

Learning About Fats

One of the most important things that helped me was a book called *Low-Fat Lies High-Fat Frauds and the Healthiest Diet in the World* by Kevin Vigilante, MD, MPH, and Mary Flynn, PhD. (LifeLine Press, A Regnery Publishing Co., 1999). There are many books out there, but I happened upon this one several years ago. It was useful in teaching me about healthy fats, unhealthy fats, and gave some good general nutrition advice. After reading it, I eliminated unhealthy and dangerous fats and began to consider including fruits and vegetables in my daily eating. At this point, in 2005, I stopped eating anything with the words *partially hydrogenated* in the ingredients. I stopped eating margarine and began to use real butter. I limited my oils to Canola and Olive Oil. Initially, I was not fanatic about this. I decided to buy and bring home Canola Oil, Olive Oil, real butter, and that's it.

While I tried to eliminate everything with the words *partially hydrogenated* in the ingredients, I was not compulsive. Remember, *MicroSteps!* I figured if it was something I ate regularly that I should eliminate it but that if it was at a party, or it was something I rarely ate, I would not make it a big deal. I tried to eat healthier without holding myself to an impossible standard of perfection.

The Food Network

Watching this television channel inspired and educated me. *The Food Network* helped immensely by teaching me how to cook in a healthier manner and it motivated me to start cooking again, instead of relying on fast food. From childhood, I'd enjoyed cooking, but I grew up in Texas and only knew how to cook heavy fattening foods. As a hobby, I'd read many cookbooks and even tried to make a few new dishes. In addition, I'd read many diet books that included numerous recipes but I never followed the diets or actually made the recipes. I had applied bits and pieces of what I'd read into my eating Routine. While I'd attended some Weight Watchers meetings back in my thirties, I'd never actually bought into healthy cooking or any specific diet plan other than counting calories.

Because of *The Food Network*, I started cooking my own meals, began to eat primarily non-processed foods, added vegetables to my daily Routine, and learned some new ways to prepare them. I discovered that when I added fruits and vegetables to my daily diet, I was less interested in unhealthy foods. One MicroStep I took was deciding to eat the healthy stuff first and then eat the junk food afterward, if I still wanted it. In the end, I did not want it because the healthy foods satisfied my cravings and filled me up. By adding vegetables and fruits, instead of taking the unhealthy foods away, less healthy foods began to disappear naturally from my daily Routine and I hardly noticed they were gone.

Watching *The Food Network*, almost daily for a while, was a great motivator. This helped me stay in touch with my goal of a healthy, average size body. It also provided my brain with constant stimulation and gave me ideas about new things to try or think about. I was learning and growing in knowledge instead of eating and getting physically larger. Learning how to cook vegetables and finding a healthy salad dressing that I liked made an enormous difference. I knew I needed to increase my intake of vegetables but until I learned how to eat them in a way that I enjoyed them, it wasn't going to happen. Finding a dressing I liked, Champagne Honey Mustard by The Silver Palate, made a huge difference in my progress toward including vegetables in my diet. It is not a diet dressing but it is healthy and you don't need a lot to get the full flavor of the dressing and the salad. Discovering the joy of a large salad with lots of raw vegetables was a big moment in my journey. I noticed my body felt better when eating vegetables. It is important to notice what makes your body feel good and what makes it feel bloated or uncomfortable.

"What Not to Wear"

The television show was both motivational and informative. Watching *What Not to Wear* caused me to want to start shopping for clothes again. I had given up on fashion and had been trying to ignore how I looked. Miserable and humiliated by my appearance, *What Not to Wear* forced me to admit this by reminding me of how tired I was of the physical pain of trying to walk and move. Consider the challenges of shopping when you're obese. As I watched the participants on the show go shopping, I remembered how difficult it was for me to shop. I'd quit shopping because I would run out of breath, my face would get all flushed, and I would become overheated and sweaty. It was not a pretty sight. Stacy London and Clinton Kelly, the stylists on the show, talked about accepting your size and dressing the body you have not the body you want.

As with my eating, I began to take MicroSteps with regard to shopping, accepting my size, and finding a way to feel better about the way I looked. I began to believe that I could be an average size again and that it did not matter if I ended up with loose skin and wrinkles. Loose skin is better than being so large you cannot function at your potential. Yes, I had worried about loose skin and wrinkles but I got past it and so can you.

Even with shopping and beginning to dress more fashionably, I had to take things one MicroStep at a time. It had to be broken down into manageable pieces so that I did not become discouraged and give up. Accepting that my size did not define me and finding a way to still love myself was an important part of my journey to end living large. Watching *What Not to Wear* played an important role in my re-entry into life in the average lane.

The First MicroSteps®

Making changes in tiny steps was the secret that prevented me from giving up. I cannot say enough about how important it was for me to take this journey slower than slow.

One of the first things I decided to do was stop eating fast food. For years, I had been working late in my private practice and then stopping for fast food on the way home. Of course, I would eat it in the car while driving. The problem with eating in the car is that you are not even looking at the food. Have you ever *really* looked at the meat in some of the fast food burgers? Not very appealing! In the beginning, I tried to stop eating the fast food altogether. But after getting off work, I was starving, and I knew there was nothing tempting waiting for me at home; I realized I just couldn't stop cold. Finally, being a good little therapist, I asked myself what I could do to end my addiction to fast food. I decided to stop eating fast food in the car. One would think this would be easy but it was very challenging. I was hungry, the food smelled good, and the French fries were right there next to me. I have to admit that it took a while but after a couple of small successes and big failures, today I no longer eat fast food. I cannot even stand the thought of it.

Another MicroStep I took was to change what I ate for breakfast. At the time, my daily breakfast Routine included three eggs fried or scrambled in two to three pats of butter, two pieces of toast with four more pats of butter, and five to eight cups of coffee. Initially, I said to myself, "I will just change one meal at a time." That seemed less overwhelming. My intention was to develop a healthy breakfast Routine and then improve what I was eating for lunch. Well, that was far too difficult. I failed miserably. So, I decided to continue eating as usual for breakfast but to eat only one piece of toast instead of two. Even that was too much for me.

After several failed attempts to eliminate one of my precious pieces of toast, I decided that if all I accomplished was removing a small half of a pat butter from one of the two pieces of toasts that I would celebrate. Okay, that small half of a pat butter did not make a difference in my weight or health at that moment; however, because my eating was so totally out of control, it was a huge step for me to say "no" to myself, a huge step for me to give up a little bit of my butter.

It worked. Over time, I reduced my large breakfast to one piece of whole grain wheat toast, one or two soft-boiled eggs, and one pat of butter. No, I do not measure the butter. Sometimes I eat oatmeal instead of eggs. Other times, I have two eggs with only one yolk. Frequently, I have peanut butter on whole grain toast and a hardboiled egg with or without the yolk. Currently, I cannot imagine eating as much for breakfast as I was eating when I stumbled upon the concept of MicroSteps. My wants have completely changed. I have new comfort zones.

In the beginning, I worked on meals during the week but continued to eat whatever I wanted on the weekend. By the time I had developed healthy eating Habits and Routines during the week, I had already started changing the weekends without trying. I believe my weekends eating Habits began to change because junk food, fast food, and overeating became less desirable after eating healthy all week.

Fruits and Vegetables

I'd never developed a taste for vegetables. Fruits were okay but I did not think of them as a food that would fill you up if you were hungry. The first MicroStep I took with vegetables and fruits was to simply buy them and bring them home. If they were not even in the house, how would I ever learn to cook or eat them? I told myself to just buy the vegetables and fruits, and take them home. It is okay if you end up throwing them away. Celebrate the fact that you brought them home. It worked. As we continue, I will share more of this story but I now eat five to six servings of fruits and vegetables daily, with generally *three* of those servings as vegetables.

There were several other MicroSteps that helped. I would cook a new dish. I began to defer gratifications, wait ten minutes before I ate the ice cream. I learned that changing one meal or one small part of a meal at a time was more successful than doing it all at once. I worked on ending my addiction to artificial sweeteners. I've learned to meet my need for sweets with a 4 oz glass of juice at night instead of ice cream. I have also discovered that fruit reduces my craving for sweets. Again, these discoveries took time and happened in MicroSteps.

Self-Discipline and Deferred Gratification

Admitting the need for self-discipline was important. The development of self-discipline as a way of life, rather than just a way to lose weight, was helpful in teaching me to defer gratification by taking MicroSteps. We make our children wait until they have finished their meal before having dessert and yet we forget that we can say "no" to ourselves. We love our children far too much to allow them to have anything and everything they want the minute they want it. We teach them to wait. We must do the same for ourselves so that we may learn to defer gratification and take MicroSteps in our journey to becoming a healthy, average size person.

Making Friends with Water

Over time, I was able to give up excessive caffeine and learn to drink water. At the beginning of my journey, I had been drinking at least a gallon of iced tea and five to ten cups of coffee daily, both loaded with artificial sweeteners. I was not drinking water.

I am please to say that I now primarily drink water. I have an average of two cups of coffee daily and an occasional iced tea. I almost never drink soda. When I am ill, to settle my stomach,

I have an occasional soda such as 7-UP (regular, never diet) which ends up to being once or twice a year. As a side note, giving up artificial sweeteners has reduced my appetite for sweets and my stomach feels better without them. I simply use sugar in moderation but rarely need it in coffee or tea. I am proud to say I've learned to like my coffee black and my tea unsweetened. That took a couple of years and several MicroSteps but I got there.

Reaching the Point Where You've "Had It" with Living Large

If you have never had a weight problem, you may find this section depressing. I understand. The fragile souls who are living with severe obesity will identify and I hope feel understood. At 315 pounds, I suffered daily from the many losses and challenges of living large. The losses are the things one has to give up because of the dysfunctional Habits, Routines, Rituals, and Traditions (HRRTs) that have been causing weight management problems. And the challenges refer to the daily struggles physically, emotionally, spiritually, and socially that we must face when we are obese, overweight, and unhappy with our body size. While any amount of weight above or below that with which you are comfortable creates problems, the extreme overweight live with severe struggles.

With so many loses and challenges it may strike others as amazing that we don't get sick and tired of it sooner, but sometimes we have to hit bottom before we've had enough. Let's look at some of the everyday losses and challenges faced by those who are living large. I know them well!

Lowered Self-Esteem

This is a major issue and a constant challenge when you are overweight. It does not mean that you have generalized low self-esteem to all areas of your life. You may feel great professionally, or have confidence as a good parent. However, deep down, when you hate what you see in the mirror, low self-esteem happens. While I had learned to love and appreciate my strengths and accept my limitations, I still felt a wave of shame because my physical presentation was so incongruent with my professional, cognitive, spiritual, and social self.

Shame and Humiliation

Shall we discuss fitting into airplane seats, booths at a restaurant, theater seats, and chairs that just do not fit? If your self-esteem can take this without feeling ashamed and humiliated, then you are a rare individual. Again, even a mentally healthy, self-confident person has limits to what they can tolerate, not to mention how much it hurts to squeeze into a chair where the arms of the seat are hurting your sides and causing pain throughout the flight, the workshop, the church service, or the movie. It hurts when the seat is too small. It hurts physically, emotionally, and you feel as though everyone notices. You experience shame and humiliation again and again.

Physical Pain

Nothing can limit your physical activities like physical pain. It hurts to walk; it hurts to get up and move. Every step hurts so you take fewer steps, often not walking unless you absolutely must. People say, "You need to exercise," without realizing how difficult it is to just take a shower and get dressed. The excessive weight lowers your physical energy, makes breathing difficult, makes it hard to put on your socks, makes it hard to stand long enough to take a shower, and robs you of precious physical, emotional, and spiritual energy. It leads to discouragement and sometimes even clinical depression. You go out with a friend, not wanting to make it all about you, but then your back hurts, your feet hurt, and finally you have to say, "Can we sit and rest for a minute." This is humiliating. How much shame can one person tolerate before experiencing a major loss of self-esteem? Many large people just give up and stop going out, stop moving, and then they get larger.

Eating is a Daily Distress

Eating causes your stomach to hurt and lowers your energy. This can happen because of eating unhealthy foods or overeating. Yet, you keep eating because you have to eat to live. Not only does overeating cause the body to feel stuffed and bloated, but junk foods cause you to feel even worse. Still, you eat junk food because you feel driven to what comforts you and you are hungry, so you do not know what else to do. You end up with low energy, stomach pain, and tremendous shame. Yes, I have been there and yes, I know.

On the positive side, once I had almost stopped eating fast foods altogether, I began to notice that whenever I *did* have a fast food cheeseburger with fries, I retained fluids, and my weight shot up two or three pounds the next day. I had an energy drop that I couldn't afford because when you're obese your energy is already low. The high fat and sodium in fast foods was making everything worse. Unbelievably, giving up fast food felt like a loss in the beginning because I truly loved those fries and cheeseburgers, though I felt much better in the long run. For me, recovery from fast food was like recovery from a drug addiction.

Shopping for Clothes

This can be a nightmare when you're overweight or obese. Today, Plus Sizes are easy to find, so one would think that even large people could shop and be stylish. Well, this is not as easy as you might think. First, there is the physical energy needed to go shopping for clothes, shoes, and accessories. Second, there is the challenge of finding clothes that are not made of Spandex or Polyester. How can one dress professionally, stylishly, and with some level of sophistication, if one cannot find clothes made of nicer fabrics, modern styles, and quality? While finding stylish Plus Size clothing might be a little easier for those who live in larger cities like New York or Los Angeles, for people who live in small towns, it is a traumatic chore.

How many times have you gone into a clothing store, with money to spend, only to find there is nothing but cheaply made clothes? The result is that you end up settling for whatever covers your body and trying to avoid looking in the mirror. This has a disastrous impact on self-esteem as well as how others perceive you.

Another unpleasant experience is going into a store, any type of store, and finding sales people who offer to help the average size customers while ignoring you. This is humiliating and a familiar experience for the large size person. One might wonder why the sales people assume that the average size person is the only one with money to spend. Also embarrassing is being patronized by a sales person who cannot wait to get away from you. You leave feeling *shame*. If you are strong enough in your self-esteem to accept that it is *their* prejudice, you are tougher than most. The majority of large people experience this humiliation frequently. Even a self-confident mentally healthy person has feelings, including the psychotherapist writing this book.

Sleep Problems

When you are obese and you try to sleep, your weight causes limbs to fall asleep, and other parts of your body, such as your back, to hurt. You end up tossing and turning throughout the night and not getting good deep sound sleep. The loss of sleep makes daily life challenging and lowers physical energy, emotional energy, and motivation in all areas.

Inhibited Social Life

Many obese people, myself included, were not always obese. It is a challenge to live large with the memories of those days when you were an average size, enjoying life, surrounded by people, and shopping for clothes. Many others, who may have been living large from childhood, cannot even muster up enough self-esteem to try starting a social life or developing social skills.

Living large greatly reduces your social life, causes your wardrobe to make you look like you do not care about your appearance, and makes you less confident around people. If you push yourself hard enough, you may continue to function and experience some professional and social success, but imagine if you had been an average size. Many obese people are not able to push themselves to that success and end up living a life much below their talents and potential.

Depression

Hopelessness and depression are mates. Trying to lose weight only to find that you gain it back and more causes you to experience a tremendous sense of hopelessness and the feeling that society does not understand. No matter which diets you try, they only give you temporary weight loss, you feel deprived, and you are unable to stick to them for the rest of your life. How profoundly discouraging it is to constantly question yourself as to why you cannot simply lose weight.

It's common for the obese person to experience clinical depression. Depression can cause overeating for comfort, sleep problems, and a severe reduction in social and physical activity. One gets caught in the cycle of dieting, regaining the weight, social and occupational humiliation, clinical depression, and repeating the cycle again and again. Depression leads to giving up socially, emotionally, and often results in isolating. The brief moments of diet success are only to be met with regaining the weight again. When you finally reach the point where you find yourself saying, *"Enough already,"* that's a good sign.

Now what?

Attending to Your Mental Health

To begin this new lifestyle, you need to be objective about what your issues are and what could interfere with making changes to the *Habits, Routines, Rituals, and Traditions* (HRRTs) that are causing you to maintain an overweight body. The journey to a healthy, average size body will be more difficult if you have not addressed issues such as severe anxiety, depression, suicidal thinking, or if you are abusing drugs or alcohol. Many life situations could sabotage your success. Some examples of these would be living in a family where you are mocked or verbally abused, living in a situation where there is domestic violence or sexual abuse, living in an environment where everyone around you abuses drugs and alcohol, or simply being in an unhappy marriage.

If you are struggling with anger issues, have chaos in your social life, or are living in a dysfunctional family that has severe problems, then you may need to seek professional help. You would be encouraged to do some work with a licensed psychotherapist as you begin your journey to a healthy, average size body. I have never met a person without issues. The wonder of MicroSteps is that they work to help resolve all kinds of issues, not only food intake.

Depression, for example, has a significant impact on eating, sleeping, and activity levels, all of which play a critical role in managing weight and physical health. If you are depressed, I encourage you to seek help from a licensed mental health professional in combination with using MicroSteps to help manage food intake.

If you have an eating disorder such as anorexia or bulimia, professional therapy can help to work on those issues as you continue down the road to a new lifestyle using MicroSteps. While the MicroSteps described in this book is not a recovery program for eating disorders, in conjunction with a medical supervision, a licensed psychotherapist, and working with a nutritionist, it could be a support. This would depend upon the severity of the eating disorder and the advice of your medical doctor and psychotherapist.

Keeping an Open Mind

The MicroSteps journey requires being open to gaining personal insight into your feelings and behaviors related to your Habits, Routines, Rituals, and Traditions (HRRTs). It is important to be objective about yourself so that you can observe and review your own behaviors, feelings, issues, and thoughts about life and food.

Qualities such as patience and the ability to be honest in how you view your own behaviors are important during this journey. For example, your body may not start to lose weight for a while; it could take months or even a year, depending on your individual issues. Patience is critical here or you will give up and return to your old ways of eating and dieting. Did you ever try to carry a cup of hot coffee across a floor with white carpet? I have and believe me I walked slowly and carefully to make sure I got to my destination without spilling my delicious coffee or spoiling the beautiful carpet. It would have been a disaster to rush to the destination (losing weight), spill the coffee (return to bad eating Habits), and ruin the carpet (gained more weight).

Determining that you will *never give up* but will work in MicroSteps toward your goal of a healthy, average size body is a gift you give yourself. The ability to celebrate yourself for what may seem to others as insignificant achievements, to feel proud when you accomplish a small change, is necessary or you will give up. Having challenges in your life does not mean that you cannot take this journey and succeed. We all have challenges. Working though them in bits and pieces, MicroSteps, is a path open to all.

Attending to Your Basic Needs

This concept is simple; you must begin at the beginning. That means you need to start at whatever point you find yourself. The basic needs for food, shelter, safety, family, and positive social support need to be in place or at least you need to be aware of these issues and start working on them—taking MicroSteps. If not addressed, they will create anxiety, driving you back to that old comfort zone of unhealthy Habits, Routines, Rituals, and Traditions overpowering the desire for change.

We often hear someone say that another person is *controlling* or has *control issues*. Well, let me tell you, *control issues* get a bad rap. Now is the time to take control of your life. It is okay to say no to someone when what he or she wants is going to cause *you* pain. It is okay to take control of what you eat, when you eat, and how what you eat is prepared. It is okay to take back the power in your social life, your economic life, your family situation, and every other aspect of your life. It is your life and you need to be the CEO, the president, the top dog in your life. In fact, it is more than okay; it is necessary, if you want to end up with a healthy, average size body. Just for the record, this is a positive kind of control. I am not talking about abusive control, such as when a husband tries to control everything the wife does and hurts her when she does not obey. That is domestic violence and it is never acceptable.

So, make sure your foundation is in place as you begin taking MicroSteps to a healthy, average size body. For example, you may need to attend to your health, finances, personal safety, clothing, friends, family, and support system. It can be very difficult to change your Habits, Routines, Rituals, and Traditions if you are struggling just to keep the day-to-day basics managed.

Does this sound difficult? It may sound that way. We all know that gaining control over weight issues is not simple. You would not believe me if I told you this would be easy. This may be challenging in the beginning, but surprisingly, it will get easier as the days pass. The journey will become your new set of Habits, Routines, Rituals, and Traditions, your new comfort zone. Remember, it took you a while to become the size you are and it will take you a while to recover your health and become a healthy, average size. Once you have started the journey, all you have to do is allow your body to catch up, as you move forward one MicroStep at a time.

Are you ready to take an honest look at your daily life, friends, family, finances, education, spirituality, and mental health so that you may choose your first MicroStep? Say you were building a house. Would you put the roof on without the foundation or the walls? No! You would start with the foundation; it is the same with this adventure to your new comfort zone.

There is no need to wait until you have a perfect life before beginning the journey to a healthy, average size body. All you need is to become aware of a couple issues and pick something that needs additional attention. Pick a small starting place. The magic of MicroSteps is that you cannot fail, as long as you start with a super tiny, very small, simple step in the beginning. Overwhelming yourself will only lead you back to comfort foods and negative HRRTs.

You are not required to keep a journal, get approval from a psychotherapist, prove you are clean and sober, keep track of calories, or anything else. No food is *off limits*. Of course, you may do anything that you decide will be helpful. It is your journey. You only need to become more aware of your issues, and begin to work on one part of a small issue. Take it slowly. Moving too quickly will cause anxiety or upset that will sabotage the journey. This is a journey for the rest of your life. It is the beginning of a new lifestyle. You will continue to grow and improve over time. Insight and awareness breeds a desire for more awareness. Awareness and a determination to change will lead you to a healthy, average size body.

Now let's move on to identifying the Habits, Routines, Rituals, and Traditions that are causing you to remain overweight and unhappy.

CHAPTER 3

Exploring Your Comfort Zones

LISTENING TO YOUR HEART CAN lead to wisdom and happiness. It helps us initiate relationships, drives us to create families, and makes us want to be with others. Listening to our hearts makes us better people, causes us to help others, to rescue animals, and to give of ourselves even when we are tired. When America listens to its collective heart, we send thousands of people into foreign countries to provide support to a people suffering after a natural disaster.

Certainly, continue listening to your heart. However, let's add a deeper awareness of what's driving that passion. Listening to your heart can get you into trouble if you listen *only* to your heart and do not engage your mind in the process. To better understand what drives you to overeat, we need to notice what drives the sadness when you hear of an abused child, what makes you angry when someone won't listen to what you have to say, or what triggers a desire to give money that you need for bills to help another person. Many people do not realize the powerful influence our personal history has on our feelings and behaviors. Deeply imbedded in our minds and hearts, the memories of lifelong Habits, Routines, Rituals, and Traditions (HRRTs for short) provide a comfort zone.

Whenever I walk into a convenience store and see those small pecan pies for a dollar on the checkout counter, I think of my dear Texas grandmother. You must know the pies I'm talking about, they're about the size and shape of a Reese's Peanut Butter Cup, unhealthy but tasty. You see, my grandmother made pecan pies for holidays when I came to visit. They were always at her house. I can remember eating pecan pie even for breakfast. Pecan pies trigger a warm feeling in my heart, make me a little sad because I miss my grandmother, and are difficult to resist. Pecan pies were a Tradition at our holiday events; they represent family and love to me. I realize it is only a pie but my heart responds with a different kind of passion. If I ever make you a pecan pie, you should know that you are loved.

I cannot even think of a pot roast without thinking of my childhood and Sunday lunches. My mother would start the pot roast cooking, we would go to church, and there it would be when we came home. The smell was divine! She always cooked the onions, carrots, and potatoes right in the pot. I can smell it now just thinking about it and I want to rush out and pick up a roast to make this weekend. There it is again, HRRTs tugging at my heartstrings.

I am telling you there is *comfort* in Habits, Routines, Rituals, and Traditions and their power is not limited to childhood experiences. How about what you had for dinner the night your husband proposed? How about that special candy bar you and your first love shared at a movie? Do you always buy a new dress for Passover dinner because your mother did that for you as a child? Do you have short hair because you've always had short hair? Do you open gifts on Christmas or Christmas Eve? Why? Was that what your parents did? Is it a Tradition or a Habit? What does it represent to you? Habits, Routines, Rituals, and Traditions with the comfort they provide are not only about food; they influence many aspects of our lives. These comfort zones are powerful.

Hopefully, you are starting to see how HRRTs influence our hearts and behaviors. Our history, blended with the present, drives us to make food choices, often without awareness of what lies beneath. This lack of awareness makes it almost impossible to choose healthier foods that support a healthy, average size body. Instead, we continue to overeat and gain weight; this causes our heart to hurt, as we feel guilty and believe we have failed.

How many times have you heard statements such as these: "We always eat that on Christmas." "I never have a birthday party without my special chocolate cake." "Mother always brings the fruit salad." "We must have that on Passover. We do every year." " We always have Easter at Aunt Jane's house. Why would we switch?"

The power of Habits, Routines, Rituals, and Traditions is not always negative. How about the Tradition of tucking your daughter into to bed with a story each night? What about the Routine of making sure you say, "I love you" to your children as you drop them off at school? Maybe you do that because that's what your mother said to you, and it feels comfortable. The power of HRRTs is pervasive in our lives, silently controlling many of our actions, choices, decisions, and beliefs.

When we abruptly abandon a comfort zone, one of the HRRTs, we experience a feeling of being a little uneasy. Most of the time we make these changes without awareness and we tolerate the discomfort. It's after we have abruptly changed several HRRTs, such as going on a diet, that we experience a feeling of stress. We may be okay in the beginning but then we struggle with a feeling of anxiety when we hit a bump in the road during a special event or crisis. The anxiety causes us to return to the old Habits, Routines, Rituals, and Traditions to put us back in the comfort zone. For some people, this may mean comfort foods but for others it could mean alcohol, drugs, unhealthy relationships, or other things that have a negative impact on their lives.

We need our Habits, Routines, Rituals, and Traditions (HRRTs). With the challenges of modern society, we need comfort zones to help calm our daily stress. Significant portions of our lives revolve around food and social eating. We receive comfort from what we eat, how we eat, when we eat, and with whom we eat. We need this comfort, identity, sense of safety, and feeling of being connected. Our HRRTs give us this and help us feel that calmness of connection to our history. For us to be able to meet those deep emotional needs, we must be able to eat whatever we want for the rest of our lives. In order to end our war with food, it makes sense then to change the negative Habits, Routines, Rituals, and Traditions that are keeping us physically unhealthy and overweight. The challenge is to do this without giving up our comfort zones, a delicate task to be sure.

Habits, Routines, Rituals, and Traditions

Defining the terms Habits, Routines, Rituals, and Traditions is the beginning of identifying negative as well as positive HRRTs. Different dictionaries defines them similarly but with slight variations. There is no need to be perfect as to the definitions or debate their slight differences. The idea here is to understand what's influencing your eating, so if you confuse a Habit with a Routine, be not dismayed. A general understanding of the definitions is good enough to get us going on our MicroStep journey. All you need to do is get the idea and increase self-awareness.

Habits, Routines, Rituals, and Traditions

For our purposes, I defined them as follows:

- **Habit** as *a behavior one repeats* so often it becomes typical and often without awareness.

- **Routine** as *a sequence of behaviors* one repeats often, without thought, predictable, and unchanging.

- **Ritual** as *an established formal behavior* one follows regularly, precisely, and often with awareness.

- **Tradition** as *handed down customs or beliefs* determining a way of life that are long established often from generation to generation.

Habits are unavoidable and are pervasive in all of our lives. A Habit is a behavior we do without awareness. Habits may include something as simple as where you put down your keys when you come home from work. It could be on which shelf you place the cheese in the refrigerator. A Habit could be how you answer your phone, how often you shave, the route you drive to work, whether or not you eat fast food after working late, what you wear on the weekend, what you eat, which news channel you watch, how you greet your children after school, and endless other things. The majority of our Habits are harmless and simply the style in which we live our lives. Some Habits are not harmless and cause us to eat badly, perhaps drink too much alcohol, or leave the house in a messy clutter that causes us to be late for work because we never put our keys in the same place. For our purposes, we are going to be looking at Habits that cause us to eat in ways that result in our becoming overweight and miserable.

As an experiment, I recently tried to change where I leave my hairbrush after I finish doing my hair each morning. All I did was to place it in a different location in the bathroom. I found myself feeling frustrated each morning when I had to reach into a different drawer for the brush. I felt distracted and ended up putting the brush back in its the original place. It seemed as though my hand was going to the original location anyway. I had to stop and remember that the brush was in the other drawer. Okay, I admit it, I am too organized, but it suits me. If you are a person who does not necessarily care about putting things in the same place, this might not bother you at all. We are all different. The point here is that even insignificant Habits are difficult to change. Changing the Habits that influence our eating is challenging but doable.

You need to become aware of your own Habits to discover which are supporting unhealthy eating. In my twenties, I had a Habit of drinking a Diet Dr. Pepper each morning, as I began teaching elementary school. Perhaps there was even caffeine addiction involved. I only know that now I do not drink sodas more than once or twice a year and I enjoy a cup or two of coffee each morning. Habits are going to change anyway. Why not make timely intentional changes that support the healthy, average size body you so greatly desire?

One way to begin this journey is to start with a Habit. You could just as easily start with a Routine, a Ritual, or a Tradition. Just pick something easy. Identify your morning Habits that influence what you eat before noon. Decide what you want your food Habits to be in the mornings. Then choose the simplest thing that you might change. Make sure it is so easy and simple, a MicroStep, that you cannot fail. Do not start with more than one MicroStep at a time. Do not begin by trying to stop having your favorite breakfast or eliminating your favorite coffee! Notice that I said, "Do not start with a favorite." That is one sure way to fail. Yes, you may need to change some of your favorite Habits later but let us begin with something easy that will give you a sense of success and power. The rest will come in good time.

Routines are unavoidable. We frequently change our Routines to meet our changing life situations. We adjust the Routine when the toddler begins preschool, when we change jobs, when we go to college, when we are married, get a divorce, or decide to take a class on Wednesday night. A Routine is as a sequence of behaviors repeated often, without thought, predictable, and generally unchanging unless something in our life changes. Routines dictate the order we do what is needed to get ready for work each day. Routines determine when we cook a meal, how we pay our bills, or where we go after work. We automatically patronize the same stores. Routines remind us when to walk the dog or to feed the cat. Because of Routines we decide what to make for dinner, where we go for fun, what television shows we watch, when to have sex, how often to meet with friends, how we study for a test, or what time the kids take their baths. Don't spend time worrying if something is a Habit or a Routine. It doesn't matter as long as you identify the behaviors that lead to eating badly.

Now, I love ice cream! I can eat ice cream almost any time. I feel the same way about pudding and flan. Having said that, at some point in my journey I decided my ice cream Routine was not supporting a healthy, average size body. In fact, it was supporting a much larger body and that body was not so healthy. At that time, I was eating three or more cups of ice cream every night just before going to bed. It was something that felt good emotionally, a soft soothing comfort, and I loved it just before bedtime. I was not fussy; I would switch hit between the flavors but looked forward to it every night. It was part of my going to bed Routine; you could even call it a Habit. Who cares? It was not working for me regardless what I call it. One thing that helped, as I struggled to get my ice cream Habit under control, was to recognize the comfort was coming from that icy-cold, smooth, sweetness in my mouth. It turned out a MicroStep that helped was to have four to six ounces of ice-cold fruit juice instead. Eventually, I did not miss the ice cream and no longer needed the juice. I tried frozen yogurt but found I ended up eating too much of it. I will tell you more about how I altered my ice cream Habit in another chapter. The point is that it was an unhealthy HRRT and it was helping to keep me obese and miserable.

Rituals are common, generally well established, and intended. They are established formal behaviors that one follows regularly, precisely, and often *with* awareness. These are not mindless acts but are behaviors that we have chosen or determined to have in our lives. We may have some of the same Rituals, as did our family of origin while growing up. Rituals may include the way we let our spouse know our needs, how we celebrate our children's birthdays, or what we do on our anniversary. Rituals help us decide where we go for a holiday dinner, what times we go to church or temple, and whether or not the family eats dinner at the table. Things such as how we prepare our children for the first day of a new school year, how we determine what to wear to a restaurant, and how we greet people are Rituals that play a role in our daily lives. Do you have a Friday night or a Sunday morning Ritual? Is the decision to shower in the morning or before bed at night a Ritual? Try to change them and the uneasiness you feel will answer the question for you.

While, Habits, Routines, and Rituals do overlap, Rituals include more awareness than does a Habit or Routine and are much more deliberate. We do these regularly, intentionally, and find them to be a comfort in that they give structure to our lives. This is fine as long as they are healthy Rituals that support a healthy, average size body. If the Ritual is to eat a double stack of pancakes with bacon and syrup for breakfast on Saturday mornings, because you've done that since you were five, that Ritual may be problematic. If the Ritual is that you always order Pizza on Friday nights, after a long workweek, so that you don't have to cook dinner, ask yourself, "Is this Ritual supporting a healthy, average size body?

As I mentioned earlier, it is not so easy to differentiate between Habits, Routines, and Rituals. Remember, it doesn't matter. Some of your behaviors may have aspects of more than one HRRT. The point is that you recognize the negative impact and take MicroSteps toward change so that you are supporting a healthy, average size body.

Traditions are deeply imbedded in our hearts, our souls, our behaviors, and our minds. Traditions are handed down as customs or beliefs that determine our way of life. We are generally aware of our Traditions. Traditions are most often passed down over generations, were the way we grew up, reflect the beliefs of our families, and go to the core of who we are in the world. They direct how we understand life, death, and dictate our basic belief systems. Traditions give us meaning and direct our way of living. Some obvious Traditions are religious beliefs, the absence of religious beliefs, ethnic customs, how we determine the relationship between men and women, our value system, what we see as right and wrong, our work ethic, how we understand people and politics, our value or absence of value regarding education, and many more.

Traditions are the most difficult to change and are likely not the primary reason we are eating badly. Having said that, I believe knowledge and awareness give you power; therefore, it is important to become more aware or cognizant of your Traditions. You may find that there is a Tradition that is causing you some problems, perhaps enough so that it becomes something you want to consider changing as you travel this road.

Again, for our goal of creating a healthy lifestyle, you do not need to label each behavior or belief perfectly as a Habit, Routine, Ritual, or Tradition. What is important is that you understand the general idea of identifying behaviors or beliefs that prevent you from having a lifestyle that supports the weight and physical health you are seeking. The HRRTs are listed in the order of Habit, Routine, Ritual, and Tradition because the Habits are the easiest to change, Routines a little more difficult, Rituals much more challenging, and Traditions the most difficult. Start with the easiest, as you are beginning to make changes.

Habits, Routines, Rituals, and Traditions define our lifestyles. The idea is to change the lifestyle first so that as you lose weight you will automatically maintain a healthy, average size body. Eat to maintain only the weight you want and eventually you will be that weight. Up until now, we have had it backwards. We lose the weight and then try to maintain the loss. We inevitably gain it back because we have not changed our lifestyle. Our HRRTs prevents our success because they are not supporting a lifestyle that maintains a healthy, average size body. If you work to maintain a lifestyle that will support a healthy, average size body, other parts of your life will inevitably become healthier.

We need comfort from Habits, Routines, Rituals, and Traditions, therefore, we need to create HRRTs that not only support a healthy, average size body but also provide comfort. We need to be able to eat whatever we want forever; healthy Habits, Routines, Rituals, and Traditions must support this. If not, we will return to unhealthy HRRTs when we need comfort. Our *wants* must change. Habits, Routines, Rituals, and Traditions are powerful. If you intentionally and slowly, in MicroSteps, implement healthy HRRTs that support a healthy lifestyle, your wants will change and you will not regain the weight.

Be Your Own Private Eye

Explore your HRRTs fully, in great depth, and in many areas for the rest of your life. That does not mean you are going to spend hours and hours thinking deeply about every behavior. It simply means you develop an automatic awareness of your

HRRTs and notice the impact they are making in your eating and in your life. Are they helping or causing problems?

Once you learn how to be aware, it is almost as easy as breathing. You just notice. Do you remember when you first learned to drive a car? You had to think of when to put your foot on the break. Once you've been driving for a while, you notice the foot is on the break but it is not a major event. There is an automatic awareness. Generally, our HRRTs are automatic and we aren't focused on them. I want you to develop an automatic awareness of the HRRTs that is as easy as breathing. Only then can you have choices as to what HRRTs you keep and what changes you determine to make. Awareness is a big step forward. In fact, it is the first step toward a healthy, average size body.

Coming up are some questions to help you develop an increased awareness of your Habits, Routines, Rituals, and Traditions so that you may begin your journey. There are endless questions you may ask yourself; the idea is to fully explore *who, when, what, where, why,* and *how* regarding everything that influences your relationship to food.

The following questions may seem like just a bunch of questions, easily read. Consider these questions as a *private investigator inside you* who is getting to know you *inside out* until it becomes clear which Habits, Routines, Rituals, and Traditions are causing you to maintain an unhealthy, overweight body. Take your time reading these. Stay with them for a while. Remember, as long as you are developing awareness, you are closer to becoming a healthy, average size person. Of course, you cannot stop with awareness; there must also be actions but awareness is the first step.

Your goal is to develop a deep level of personal awareness. This cannot be done solely with pen and paper, quickly writing the answers to a few questions. While you might want to do some writing, you need to think. Think briefly, think deeply, think while going about your day, think while you are doing anything, and become more aware of everything. Consider these questions as one considers a *thought for the day*. Take one or maybe two questions a day (or for a week) and keep them in your mind as you live your daily life. See what you notice. Do not assume that you already know all the answers. There is a deeper level of awareness, I promise. It doesn't matter which question you start with; pick the question that *jumps out at you*. Add your own questions.

This is *your* journey. It is your wisdom and increasing knowledge of yourself that will take you to a healthy, average size body. Okay, I know you are thinking. Lack of wisdom resulted in a weight problem. Well, fear not; your increased awareness of your Habits, Routines, Rituals, and Traditions will provide the tools you need to take your wisdom to a higher level. You may feel like you're walking in the dark at first, but it will become easier in MicroSteps.

The next page(s) should take a while to absorb. Glance over them quickly, get the idea, and then choose one or two questions. Once you feel you have completely explored those two, pick another question—or two. You will find your Habits, Routines, Rituals, and Traditions in the outcome of your exploration and that awareness will guide you on your journey. You may find yourself returning to these questions repeatedly to help guide you on your way.

Relationship to Food

- Who prepares my food?
- Where do the bulk of my meals occur?
- When do I eat the majority of my daily calories?
- What factors in my environment influence my eating choices?

Career, Work (or School)

- Do I skip breakfast on workdays?
- How does my work influence my eating?
- What do I eat when I am at work or school?
- Does everyone at work order fast food or go out to eat daily?

Social Life and Relationships

- What foods remind me of my childhood?
- How do my family members and friends eat?
- At what social events do I end up eating badly?
- Do I eat when hungry or when it is socially expected?

Physical Activities

- Where do I get physical exercise?
- Are my social activities ever physical?
- How much do I know about how to exercise?
- Do my friends enjoy being physically active?

Style and Self Care

- How much sleep do I get each night?
- Do I get up, get dressed, and get out every day?
- How does the way I look impact my social activities?
- Does the way my shoes feel affect my willingness to take a walk?

Feelings and Emotions

- How does being upset affect my eating?
- Is food always a part of my celebrations?
- What do I eat when sad, anxious, or depressed?
- What happens to my eating when I am lonely or bored?

Intellect and Knowledge

- What kind of books do I read?
- What do I do to increase my knowledge?
- What have I learned about nutrition and healthy eating?
- How many hours a day do I watch television? What do I watch?

Daily Tasks and Duties

- How do I determine what time to eat my meals?
- Do I get too busy to eat all day and then end up overeating at night?
- Do I have an unhealthy snack at work or school just because it is break time?
- Does taking care of family dictate my food choices?

Developing a deep awareness of your Habits, Routines, Rituals, and Traditions is an ongoing process that must continue so that your insight continues to grow and evolve throughout your life. When you feel you are making an excuse for a moment of unhealthy eating, ask yourself, "Is there a HRRT that was responsible for the unhealthy choice?" If the answer is yes, you have the perfect opportunity to explore an unhealthy HRRT that is not supporting your healthy, average size body.

Think about how your HRRTs have changed dramatically over the years. They automatically change each year as you enter a new grade in school, when you go to college, when you get married, after a break-up with a lover, when you have children, or when a loved one dies. Change is inevitable and that means that the Habits, Routines, Rituals, and Traditions can and do change intentionally, automatically, with thought, without thought, easily, with great difficulty, and often. With that in mind, let us look at how the process actually works.

Take Action with MicroSteps®

- Make the Changes in MicroSteps.
- Avoid Creating Panic and Anxiety.
- Create Intentional HRRTs that will Support a Healthy, Average Size Body.

The first thing I did in trying to reach a healthy weight was to identify a behavior or Habit that was supporting my unhealthy, overweight body. The first behavior I chose to address was that of getting off work late and eating fast food in the car on the way home. This would occur around four nights a week between 8PM and 10PM. After eating fast food, I would then go home and go to bed. One could even argue that this was a Routine. It does not matter; what matters is that it was keeping me overweight and unhealthy.

At the time, I did not realize that I had started a process; I had not even thought about the HRRTs or MicroSteps. I was only trying to stop a behavior or Habit that was preventing weight loss. I was trying to diet. I thought that if I could only stop eating fast food, I could make progress. I knew that ending my addiction to fast food would be difficult, so I decided to take it in small steps. The first thing I did was to stop eating the fast food in the car and make myself wait until I got home to eat. It took about two years of struggling to accomplish this. It finally worked and one day I noticed that I did not even think about eating the fast food in the car. I did not realize it at the time, but my lifestyle was changing in a way that would eventually support the healthy, average size body I was seeking.

An author friend mentioned to me that she put the fast food in the trunk of her car while driving home. This prevented her from nibbling at the "absolutely heavenly smelling" fries that she'd bought for her husband and not for herself. That sounds like a fabulous idea! I say, "Do whatever works!" It is your journey and you must creatively find your way. Perhaps it would not have taken me so long to stop eating the fast food in the car had I thought of this trick.

Once I stopped eating fast food in the car, I decided to try to work on eliminating fast food altogether. This was significantly more difficult but eventually worked. I had to make small goals and take MicroSteps. Some of these MicroSteps included:

- Only eat fast foods at restaurants that do not use trans fats. This was a major step in improving my physical health.

- Reduce the amount of my order. Going from two burgers and two orders of fries to one burger and one order of fries was a challenge at first.

- Order the small size fries and sodas.

- Order the burger and fries but have bottled water instead of soda.

- Limit fast food to twice a week, then eventually once a week, then once a month...

- Eventually, I limited fast food to only *one* drive through restaurant because that restaurant seemed to be the closest to "healthy." It really wasn't healthy but at the time that made sense to me and helped me move forward.

Be not misled. Each step took months, some a couple of years, and was difficult. It was also critical that I acknowledged each small success. I celebrated every time I made it home without eating fast food in the car or without buying fast food at all. There were times I called a friend to talk me *past* the fast food restaurant on my way home. You must celebrate each small success and mentally connect that success to eventually being a healthy, average size person. It is not about being on a diet but about changing your lifestyle. If you are a fast food junky, as I was, then this is a major Habit, Routine, and/or Ritual for you to change.

One thing that helped me conquer my fast food Habit was making sure that I had something good to eat waiting for me at home after work each day. Acknowledging how tired I am after a long workday was critical in helping me eliminate the negative Habit/Routine of fast food. You see you cannot just take away a negative HRRT; you must replace the negative HRRT with a positive HRRT. My new HRRT is that I have great, tasty, healthy foods waiting for me at home each day after work. I look forward to going home, eating foods that make me feel good, and find that I am not even thinking about the fast food. Initially, I had things like frozen dinners, fruit, and the ingredients needed for salads waiting at home. Eventually, I learned to cook on the weekends, making foods that I could freeze to use later in the week. The Bonus Chapter at the end of this book has some of these recipes. It was important for me create the Habit of always having tasty and healthy food at home.

Handling Impatience

At some point, I became aware of what seemed like an endless list of HRRTs that were causing me to continue to be overweight. I wanted to address and change all of them immediately. I desperately wanted to be thin and look beautiful again and I did not want to wait. Once I understood the process, it was not easy to limit myself to one MicroStep at a time until I finally had changed enough of my bad Habits, Routines, Rituals, and Traditions so that my body began to lose weight.

Part of the challenge is to manage the urge to move too quickly. I let people around me think that I did not care about my weight and that I was not trying to lose weight. I felt that no one would understand my turtle's pace. Privately celebrating my small successes helped me move forward and increased my patience. To focus only on that which one has *not* accomplished results in feeling like a failure and subsequently leads one to fail.

MicroSteps based on awareness of the negative HRRTs that have been causing you to continue in unhealthy overeating give you power. This is not a diet; you don't count calories, follow a bunch of rules, or avoid certain foods. This is a journey in your mind and in your heart. The power is in your head via knowledge and awareness. The journey is one of heart and mind that helps your behaviors change so that you automatically begin to eat in a way that allows your body to become a healthy, average size.

While I was working to develop a Habit/Routine that would support a healthy satisfying breakfast, I celebrated each tiny step forward, even if all I accomplished, as mentioned earlier, was removing a small half of a pat of the four large pats of butter on my two pieces of toasts and three eggs. I celebrated and that celebration led to more successes. Success begets success, regardless of how small the step forward. I knew that I was working toward eating a healthy breakfast. I knew that I wanted to lose weight and be a healthy, average size person. I decided to take MicroSteps and allow myself to make progress that did not create anxiety or cause me frantically to go back to the comfort foods supported by unhealthy HRRTs.

It worked! The weight loss has been slow, two to four pounds a month. I don't think about food all the time, don't feel as though I am on a diet, and know I can do this forever. At some point, when I reach the size I want to remain, I will figure out what I need to eat to continue to stay that size. Right now, I am thrilled with the journey. It is like being a traveler. I know

I am on the road and from time to time, I will check the map to make sure I get to my destination. I am taking responsibility for my knowledge and awareness; I trust my brain to be able to figure out the rest of the journey. You can do this too.

Starting with MicroSteps®

Think of it this way: People generally eat three meals a day, perhaps one or two snacks, and have to make the decision to eat at home or to eat out. When you go on a diet, you generally attack all of these at once. MicroSteps allow you to choose a small starting place, to pick a meal, a part of a meal, to cook, or not cook. With MicroSteps, you may decide your goal is to eliminate an unhealthy food or add into your daily eating something healthy like a vegetable. Either way, you are making changes. You may decide to start by limiting which restaurants you patronize, changing how much of a specific food you allow (notice I did not say eliminate), changing what you drink at a certain meal, or start by eating healthy for only one hour a day. It does not matter where you start. Just start. Start simple, with something easy, so you have a good chance of succeeding. Here are just two examples as to how you might begin.

Example One:
- Pick a meal and determine to make that meal always healthy.
- Evaluate what you generally eat for that meal.
- Establish where you eat that meal. Does that need to change?
- Identify who prepares that meal. Does that need to change?

- Ask what influences your choices for that meal.

- Look at what changes might be helpful in making this meal healthier.

- Decide which one MicroStep (very small part) of that meal you can change (maybe one less dinner roll, maybe a half teaspoon of sugar instead of a whole teaspoon, maybe one pork chop instead of two, maybe where you eat the meal, maybe who prepares the meal).

- Make sure the change is small, easy, and likely to lead to success. Identify the smallest, tiniest, least anxiety producing change that you can make.

- Reassure yourself: It does not matter how small the change. This is only the beginning.

- Begin to try to make that tiny MicroStep of change daily.

- Celebrate each time you succeed with your Micro-Step of change.

Example Two:
- Determine that you are drinking, for example, too much coffee. Adjust the steps for any beverage or food.

- Decide what you would like to be drinking instead. (Let's say it is water.)

- Make sure you have the water available at all times.

- Continue to drink the coffee but drink 2-6 ounces of water before each cup of coffee.

- Evaluate what you are putting in your coffee, if anything.

- Is there too much artificial sweetener? Too much sugar or cream?

- Would you like to change what you put in the coffee?

- Make sure the change is small, easy, and likely to lead to success. Identify the smallest, tiniest, least anxiety producing change that you can make.

- Maybe you can go an extra fifteen minutes before having the second cup of coffee.

- Begin to try to make that tiny MicroStep of change daily.

- Celebrate each time you succeed with your Micro-Step of change.

I can imagine that some of you might be thinking the process is too slow and that you do not have months or years to lose weight and get to a healthy, average size quickly. I understand that feeling; we all want to be an average size yesterday! Just remember, time is going to pass regardless of what you are eating. You will gain, lose, or stay the weight you are. Has abrupt dieting worked for you in the past? Did you lose? Did you regain the weight? What harm is there in beginning to change your unhealthy HRRTs slowly? What will happen if you go on another abrupt diet? What will happen if you do nothing? Most people gain weight slowly over time. What will your weight be this time next year, if you begin taking Micro-Steps to change the unhealthy Habits, Routines, Rituals, and Traditions that caused your weight issues in the first place?

Each time you have a tiny success, celebrate in your heart. Be proud of yourself; be extremely proud! Pat yourself on the back. Reducing food intake even by a couple of fries or a half serving of pasta is a success. When you do not feel you have succeeded, say to yourself, "No problem, I am still moving forward." Immediately, continue your journey. If necessary, make the change easier or smaller. Find a way to succeed.

Continue to focus on a tiny MicroStep of change. As that change becomes easy and natural, pick a new MicroStep on which you can work. Celebrate that you have identified a MicroStep and that you are working on it. It does not matter how small the changes you make are, only that you make changes. One change will lead to another. Before you know it, you have a new Habit, Routine, Ritual, or Tradition to support your healthy, average size body. Amazingly, you are only eating the amount of food required to sustain a healthy, average size body. You can do it!

CHAPTER 4

Family, Friends, Feelings

RECENTLY, I ARRIVED AT WORK to learn that a colleague of mine had died in her sleep. That day I was facing a schedule of back-to-back psychotherapy appointments with patients who had troubles of their own. When my first appointment arrived, all I could think of was my last conversation with my colleague. She had grandchildren that she would not get to see grow up. One of her daughters was expecting another baby. It was sad. I wanted to cancel the rest of my appointments so I could be with my feelings but these were patients who needed to have their sessions that day.

With difficulty, I got through the day and was finally in my car driving home. I remembered all the years that the nearest fast food restaurant would have been an immediate source of comfort. I had not eaten fast food for well over a year. As I drove past several fast food places, I felt some of the old longings; I wanted to stop and eat my sadness away. I was exhausted. I told myself that I deserved the comfort of an easy meal. Then I remembered that what I really deserved was to feel healthy and become an average size. I also deserved the opportunity to be with my feelings and to process the day; drowning them in fast food would distract from that moment. I made it home without fast food and spent some time pondering the sadness of a life ended too soon.

Given the circumstances and my feelings, I was surprised that I had not stopped for the fast food. A week later, reflecting on the experience, I realized that my Habits, Routines, Rituals, and Traditions had truly changed. The new HRRTs were powerful enough to get me safely home on a sad day without stopping for fast food. Now, that was worth celebrating!

It is impossible to count the times I have heard someone blame overeating on being upset, depressed, anxious, angry, PMS, or even feeling happy. Emotions do and will continue to play a role in what we eat. This is not always a bad thing but we need to make sure that emotions are not sabotaging healthy eating.

Since our emotions do influence our eating, we need to look at how we manage them. You cannot fix the problem until you know what isn't working and what needs changing. We must ask ourselves, "Why do my emotions cause me to overeat?"

One reason is that we are often told to, "suck it up," "let it go," "don't say anything," or "don't rock the boat." It is difficult to cope with emotions and stressors successfully without the proper skills. If your family was one that covered things up rather that talk about *the elephant in the room*, then you may not know how to successfully deal with emotions. So often, people are all about keeping the equilibrium and avoiding what they are feeling.

How many times have you been deeply upset but just sat down to dinner, looked at your food, and ignored everything around you as you shoved the food in without even tasting it? It happens all the time. To determine what skills are missing, you must take an honest look at how your emotions are managed.

There are endless emotions that human beings experience. Here, I will be addressing four basic emotions: happy, sad, fear and anger. We'll use these four emotions as examples that provide us with a roadmap. Once you know how to identify and manage these emotions, you will likely be able to manage other emotions as well.

Four Emotions

1) Happy—*pleasure, contentment, satisfied, elated, excited, pleased, glad, joyful, cheerful, blissful, ecstatic, delighted, jovial, on cloud nine.*

Why do positive emotions require coping skills? Often we use positive situations or emotions as cause to go out and celebrate. We use these moments as reasons to overeat, drink too much alcohol, stay up too late, spend too much money, and say or do things later regretted.

Is there a way of celebrating that does not result in regrets? Of course, but that requires being able to respond to the situation from a place of comfort with oneself, one's family, and with friends. To celebrate without abusing food, alcohol, and drugs requires that one be comfortable with the intimacy of conversation and sharing emotions. To increase your comfort level with intimate conversation requires learning to observe your feelings in the moment. It requires that we learn to observe the other person in the moment as well. Intimacy is a two-way conversation or experience and is the outcome of responding rather than reacting without thinking.

Does one have to resolve to never drink alcohol or over-eat to be able to manage one's emotions in a healthy manner? No, that's not what I am saying. However, one must be able to make a choice. There is a big difference between responding to a celebratory moment by choosing to eat or drink differently than your usual way versus reacting impulsively or *going for it* without thinking. Responding leaves you in control and making a choice; reacting impulsively leaves you powerless over your emotions and out of control.

To be clear here, I am not talking about deciding to abuse alcohol or addictive drugs; that is a different issue entirely. I am talking about deciding that at the special event you will eat differently than your usual healthy way of eating and return to your healthy eating HRRTs immediately after the event. Making a decision thoughtfully to eat differently than usual puts you in charge of deciding exactly what you are going to eat. Deciding to have cake at the wedding, eat ribs and fries at the barbeque, or enjoy pizza at your daughter's birthday party is different than being in such an out-of-control celebratory mood that you are not even aware of what you are putting in your mouth.

That out-of-control celebratory behavior generally leads to guilty feelings. After out of control eating, we often end up on a downward slide, eat more, feel depressed, and return to our old comfortable HRRTs that got us into trouble in the first place. Your new HRRTs are fragile; it will take time for them to mature and become deeply imbedded in your heart. Give them the time they need to grow. Protect them by responding thoughtfully and with awareness even when you are happy and going for the fun.

2) Sad—*depressing, gloomy, miserable, cheerless, heartbreaking, distressing, heartrending, unhappy, grief, sorrow, regrettable, pitiable, dull, depressed.*

It is not only okay but it is necessary to cry. It is important to express your feelings of sadness. We must learn to be in the moment with the sadness and allow ourselves to feel uncomfortable. That does not mean we need to burst into tears out in public and draw unwanted attention to ourselves but we do need to express our feelings in a safe place and with a safe person.

If we hide the feelings of sadness inside, we end up overeating or drinking alcohol to drown them. Alcohol is a depressant. When you use alcohol to drown your sorrows, your sorrows increase and so does the alcohol consumption. People tend to either eat too much or stop eating when they are depressed—neither of which is supportive of getting you to that goal of a healthy, average size.

Just because feelings are unpleasant does not mean they are bad, wrong, or that we are unstable. We have evolved into a society that acts as though we are supposed to feel calm, comfortable, and always together to be mentally healthy. This is simply not true. Feelings are just feelings and when we do not honor them, they come out in negative ways. They drain our energy and reduce our motivation, preventing us from taking positive action.

Allowing depression or sadness to take charge of our eating and alcohol consumption leaves us feeling powerless and reactive. We need to respond to depression by taking charge of our eating, sleeping, and activity levels. This requires self-discipline and making sure to attend to our HRRTs. If we have developed healthy Habits and Routines of what, when and how we eat, of when and how many hours we sleep, of a positive social life, and have a physical activity schedule then we are more likely to be able to use these healthy Habits or Routines to help us get through the difficult times.

Sadness or depression has a powerful impact on eating, sleeping, and activity levels; that includes physical as well as social activity. We need to share our feelings in a safe way and this requires trust and comfort with intimate conversation.

3) Fear—*anxiety, terror, dread, horror, fright, panic, alarm, trepidation, apprehension, worry, concern, nightmare, phobia, afraid, frightened, unpleasant feeling of anxiety, apprehension, fear of being emotionally hurt, fear of being abandoned, fear of being embarrassed.*

Fear or anxiety can be immobilizing, causing you to stop living your life and turn to overeating, substance abuse, sleeping too much, or isolation for comfort. This of course leads to depression and feeling as though your life is completely out of your control. The important thing to remember about anxiety is that once you give into it, it grows. The first time you have a fear reaction or a panic attack you are likely reacting to a situation that has caught you off guard or frightened you. After that, there is a tendency to connect anxiety or fear to every similar situation. If you were embarrassed while grocery shopping, you associate grocery shopping with panic and embarrassment. You then avoid grocery shopping. The problem is that the anxiety or fear gets worse every time you avoid something. This is because you're anticipating the worse and your body gives you what you expect.

Panic creates more panic; worry creates more worry. Giving in to anxiety creates more anxiety. It is a vicious cycle. The answer is to learn to tolerate your feelings, in MicroSteps, without flooding yourself. The flooding happens when we force ourselves to move too quickly. Talk to yourself by saying positive statements such as: "This will pass." "I can do this." "I may feel anxious but the anxiety will be gone in a few minutes."

The danger with panic, fear, or anxiety is that people often turn to food (or addictive drugs and alcohol) for comfort. Often people isolate to avoid the feelings or end up depressed and reacting to the feelings rather than coping with the discomfort. Learning new Habits, Routines, Rituals, and Traditions to reduce the uncomfortable feelings and take control gives you back your power.

Perhaps, you're wondering if you need to seek professional support from a psychotherapist or psychiatrist. As a rule of thumb, consider the severity of the depression, anxiety, or anger. If you're feeling suicidal or you're unable to move forward in your life, then you might want to seek help. There's no shame in talking with a mental health professional and it might make the journey easier.

4) Anger—*annoyed, insulted, inflamed, irritated, fuming, mad, livid, irate, heated, cross, furious, incensed, enraged, outraged, infuriated.*

When people experience hurt feelings, fear of being shamed, fear of humiliation, fear of being disrespected and do not know what to do with those feelings, they will often put on the mask of anger. Anger is not a primary emotion. It is a cover-up emotion most often made up of unresolved hurt and fear.

Beneath anger is often a deficit in empathy, a lack of respect for the other person, or low self-esteem. Generally, this comes from how one learned to manage feelings and respond to other people during childhood and adolescence.

Another cause of anger can be absence of communication. If you have something to say and you just stuff it inside yourself, you end up with resentment. Resentment becomes anger. It bottles up and eventually boils over and spills out onto those you love.

Anger may be expressed in words, passive aggressive actions, or violence. Passive aggressive anger is subtle but can be hurtful to relationships. Passive aggressive anger behaviors include doing something just to annoy someone, being late to get even, or avoiding calling someone back. There are many other ways to be passively aggressive with your anger.

So, what do you do about anger? Explore the true feelings such as hurt or fear that are *beneath* the anger. Talk with others before the anger has a chance to build. Consider the other person's side of the story and have empathy for their situation or feelings. Consider what Habits, Routines, Rituals, Traditions are supporting the anger mindlessly and become aware of changes that might help. This is an area where professional help might be needed if the anger has become violent or out of control.

Learning to be Comfortable with Intimacy

I will bet you think this is going to be a discussion about sex. While sex is certainly part of intimacy, it is only a part. Surprised? Join the club; I would guess that the majority of people hear the word intimate and assume it relates to sex. Have you ever had sex with someone and felt the person did not know you at all? Intimacy includes a knowing and sharing; it is much more than simply being close physically.

Intimacy is about exchanging detailed personal information with another person, a familiarity, closeness, an understanding, and sharing. It is being able to tolerate the easy-to-hear as well as the more difficult to hear feelings, thoughts, ideas, and stories of another person. It is about being able to share the same about you with that other person.

Often these days we hear someone say *"TMI,"* meaning *too much information.* We live in a society of people who experience discomfort and anxiety when they find themselves in a conversation about the body and the bodily functions, about someone feeling upset or sad, about someone having a crisis, about someone not *having it together.* We expect others and ourselves to put on the face of *"I'm fine"* and to ignore our humanity. Let's face it: We all go to the toilet, brush our teeth, or have laughed or coughed so hard we peed on ourselves (and tried to hide it). We have all gotten our feelings hurt when someone said something unkind. Too often we are trying to prevent anyone from seeing our humanity or prevent ourselves from seeing theirs.

So often, we do not really look at each other, hear what another person is saying, or think about what someone is going through. We are like children in a sandbox playing with our own toy and never interacting with the other child. We are alone in the crowd and lonely in our world of emotions.

In my own situation, after losing the first fifty pounds, most people started to notice it. Often, they would ask politely if I had lost weight, usually adding something nice about how I was dressing or looking. It was fun at first. I became excited to hear what some specific friends and colleagues had to say because of experiences we had shared over the years.

I was especially interested in one friend who several years earlier had offered me unwanted advice on weight loss. Yet when I saw her again after losing fifty pounds, she said nothing. I was puzzled, until I realized that she never truly looked at me when we were together. That started me on a little people watching experiment. I noticed that frequently people do not really look at each other.

I began to look closely at other people. I noticed what they had on, the details of their outfits, the shapes of their bodies, and the imperfections that we all have. I also noticed there were some people in my life who were beautiful and dressed nicely; I had not even noticed how good they looked until now. As a therapist, I had been listening to stories, giving empathy, observing body language and faces, but I had not been looking at the physical person. We need to look at each other. This little experiment increased my self-esteem, as I realized that the real people in my life were beautiful, fat, thin, bumpy, dumpy, lean, wrinkled, sophisticated, fashionable, unfashionable, imperfect, and not so much like the folks who walk the red carpet. Intimacy includes looking at each other and accepting what you see.

None of us has it *together* all the time. Keeping people at arm's length and acting as though we are fine when we are not gets us into trouble. When we fake having it together, we end up feeling so desperate to comfort our hidden fears that in the end no one really knows us and we are ultimately alone. That drives us back to the unhealthy eating for comfort and back into depression.

It is critical to have intimacy with another person. This does not have to be a lover or spouse; it could be a good friend. It is not only about sexual intimacy; it is about sharing who you are with another human being and accepting who he or she is as well. You do not have to go around spilling your guts to everyone you talk to; just share your feelings with those you trust to love you.

Choose one or two people you feel you can trust and begin, slowly, in MicroSteps. Share the easiest parts first and build; listen to what they share and your trust will grow. Try not to judge yourself or the other person too harshly. Don't tell the other person how to fix a problem, unless asked. There is a lot to gain by simply listening and sharing without getting into problem solving or advice giving.

Observing Your Own Feelings in the Moment

Have you ever gone to lunch with a friend, feeling great, but by the time lunch was over you felt that something just went wrong; yet, you could not explain why you felt that way? Did you ever get up in the morning feeling good and then after your spouse and the kids were gone you felt anxious? Were you able to identify when the feelings changed or why they changed?

Observing your feelings the moment they happen is a learned skill. It may take some practice to get good at it but it is definitely doable. It is important. Being aware of what you are feeling *when* you are feeling it, gives you the opportunity to do something about it before it grows into a problem that causes you to feel driven to unhealthy comfort food or some other dysfunctional Habit, Routine, Ritual, or Tradition.

Observing your feelings *in the moment* is simple to describe but difficult to put into practice. You start by listening to your own body. When we have a feeling of sadness, anxiety, discomfort with a conversation, insecurity, anger, frustration, or fear our bodies actually experience something. You may feel something in your stomach or have tension in your arms or shoulders. You may find yourself distracted, be unable to concentrate, start driving faster or slower than usual, become unusually irritable with family members, or find yourself avoiding your usual activities. The idea here is to notice your behaviors and the physical feelings in your body.

How many times have you ended a conversation with someone, as I mentioned earlier, only to find yourself feeling uneasy afterwards or perhaps the next day—and not sure why? Do you find yourself thinking, "I wish I had said this or that?" Since you did not notice what you were feeling *in the moment*, you missed the opportunity to respond and ended up feeling uneasy. Did it distract you from your normal activities or ruin your day? It has happened to the all of us.

As I said, it is a *learned* skill. You *can* learn how to observe your feelings in the moment. In the beginning, just try to identify the feelings. You may not figure out the feeling until a day or two later but do not worry. You can still go to the person and talk about how you were feeling. This is the first MicroStep.

Once you are able to clarify for yourself what you are feeling, begin to try to catch the feeling *the moment it happens*. When you are able to do that, then try to express your thoughts about your feelings as they are happening. Expressing your feelings *in the moment* helps prevent them from becoming problems that upset your day, cause dysfunction in relationships, or lead to comfort eating. The more you practice this skill over time, the easier it will become.

Observing the Feelings of Others in the Moment

The idea here is to know what you are feeling, while at the same time realizing that the other person has reacted to something that you said or did. You will know this by the person's body language, a change in attitude, a facial expression, an abrupt change in conversation, and subtle changes in the person's facial movements. Notice how the person is breathing, the eye contact, the speed at which he or she is speaking, and how they respond to you.

While it is important to feel that the person is listening and understanding what you are saying, it is equally important to realize that you have triggered something in the other person. Sometimes the other person is so distracted by their own reactions that they cannot hear what you are saying. This may be because they are unable to observe their own feelings in the moment. This is the time to stop talking about the issue and ask the person how *they* are feeling about what you are saying or doing.

One of my best friends, Marie, is a little on the shy side. We often go to lunch. She is not fussy and will usually ask me to suggest the place. I remember more than once suggesting a restaurant, Marie telling me that sounded good, and then seeing her look away. Whenever she did this, I knew it was time for me to double-check and find out how she *really* felt. Often, she would admit that she had eaten that type of food just the day before or that she would rather eat somewhere else.

There is freedom in being able to tolerate intimate conversations and being able to process the good, the bad, the ugly, and travel through the muck until you get to common ground. I never said all intimate conversations would be comfortable. I just said they are necessary to help you manage your emotions and to thus avoid that race back to unhealthy HRRTs and old comfort foods.

What does this have to do with managing your weight? Everything! We need people in our lives. We respond and react to our relationships with one another. If we do not deal with our relationships and keep them healthy, we end up eating around the issues and our old negative Habits, Routines, Rituals, and Traditions take over.

Feeling the Feelings

Why not just ignore one's emotions and decide to eat healthy regardless of the mood or life situation in which you find yourself? People have been trying to do this for years; it generally does not work. If it did, more people would be able to maintain a lifestyle that supports healthy eating and weight management. The people who struggle the most with emotional eating may be those who are more sensitive to their feelings. Perhaps they are the artist types, the creative sorts, or maybe they are the people who are struggling with deeper issues or baggage from the past. Those who are more cognitive, driven by logic, or less responsive to their own emotions, may be able to put feelings and mood aside and eat only what they determine to be healthy. Then again, perhaps some of the people whose food choices are not driven by their mood are actually the people who have resolved their emotional issues and dealt with the baggage of the past.

Getting Over the Baggage from the Past

It is my observation, after providing psychotherapy for hundreds of patients, that most people have some type of baggage from the past. While we all have different histories and life experiences, we share the same emotions. We all experience basic emotions such as *happy, sad, angry, hurt, joy, fear, glad, anxious,* and many others. Our life history and experiences play a large role in determining the skills we develop to cope with those emotions. Do not be dismayed, however, if you come from a background that has left you with few skills for coping with emotions and stress. For most people, these skills can be learned and once learned will impact life in a positive way. This is a case where knowledge is your most powerful tool.

If you come from a difficult childhood, have a dysfunctional family, have suffered from domestic violence, have had to cope with losses, have been betrayed in love, were the victim of a crime, and have been unable to get past these things, you are not alone. Many people have suffered as well; there is help. Depending on your level of recovery, you may want to get into some professional counseling to help you get past these or other issues. Your goal of having a healthy, average size body may depend upon your willingness to resolve some of these issues.

Responding Rather than Reacting

This may be the most important of all the emotional management skills. A *reaction* is something you say or do without thinking. A reaction is impulsive. A *response* is something you say or do after giving it some thought—making sure that the words or actions reflect who you are and what you want to communicate.

There are times when we need to say what we are feeling *in the moment* to clarify something or nurture a relationship. There are other times when our feelings are intense and need a bit of tending to before we share them.

In the case of intense feelings, stop and think before you say or do something. Give yourself a few minutes, an hour, or a day before you say something hurtful to another person, eat something you know you will regret eating, purchase an expensive item that you cannot afford, or allow impulsive *knee-jerk* reactions to take over. This is called deferring gratification. It just means that you need to make yourself wait, gather your thoughts, calm down, determine how you want to respond, and then respond thoughtfully.

When we *react* instead of *respond* to a situation, we run the risk of over-reacting. In the moment that we react, we may experience relief because we get our feelings out. However, by deferring gratification and taking the time to determine how you want to respond, you are teaching yourself to manage your HRRTs with awareness as well as improving your relationships with friends and loved ones.

Here it is. We must learn to respond to our feelings thoughtfully and to share these feelings with others. If not, we will continue to return to old Habits, Routines, Rituals, and Traditions that lead to eating unhealthy comfort foods. When we manage our emotions in a healthy way, it is easier to manage our eating and our relationships reap the benefits of being healthier and fuller. Life becomes easier and the journey more clear.

PART TWO

Journey to a Healthy, Average Size Body

CHAPTER 5

Shop, Cook, Eat

REJOICE! YOU ARE NOT ON A DIET. However, there is work to do and *ignorance is definitely not bliss.* If you are waiting for me to tell you how to eat to lose weight, you might as well put the book down now and ask for a refund. There are endless numbers of diet books on the market; but if you plan to eat to support a healthy, average size body, without relapse, it has to be your own. You must find your own way. You must create your own eating Habits, Routines, Rituals, and Traditions. They must be a part of who you are for the rest of your life.

Having said that, I will try to point you in a healthy direction, but you need to commit to learning about nutrition, cooking, exercise, and maintaining good mental health if you want to find your own way to your own comfort zone. Whether you hire a chef, go out to eat, or cook for yourself does not matter; you need to be the one determining what goes into your body and you cannot do that without knowledge of food and nutrition.

The truth is, one cannot lose weight or maintain a healthy, average size body without eating a balanced diet. That means including foods from all the basic food groups, avoiding bad fats, limiting white flour, and using sugar sparingly. I know that's difficult to hear. Please do not stop reading. Reality is your friend; read on! Knowledge is the power you need in order to reach that goal of a healthy, average size body. How can you know which Habits, Routines, Rituals, and Traditions to change, if you do not even know what to eat?

We must eat in proportion to the energy required to keep our body functioning. Eat more than the amount needed to keep the body functioning and you will gain weight. Eat less than the body needs to function and you will lose weight. Eat large amounts of bad fats or lots of sugary foods and you will develop other health issues. I am not a doctor or a nutrition-ist but this is just common sense. Most of us already know the above or at least have some idea of the concepts. It is that simple and that complex.

The following information is critical if you want to achieve your goal of becoming a healthy, average size person. It is basic and common knowledge amongst many of those folks who do maintain healthy, average size bodies. This is what they know and apply to their regular eating Habits, Routines, Rituals, and Traditions.

It is not everything you need to know but it is a beginning. The rest is what you will need to get out and learn via books, television, websites, college classes, workshops, or by whatever means suits you. What I am sharing comes from many years of my own reading, watching television, surfing websites, col-lege classes, and trying to figure things out. I am not an expert when it comes to nutrition but think of reading the information below as a first MicroStep toward gaining knowledge. I hope this little taste will trigger a craving for more.

Proteins (animal sources, vegetable sources)

Protein comes from meats (poultry, fish, beef, and pork), eggs, and dairy products. It also comes from nuts and legumes, such as seeds, lentils, and black beans. Protein is important in that it takes care of the tissues in your body including your muscles, organs, and immune system that are made mostly of protein. Your body uses protein to make hemoglobin and build up cardiac muscles; we need protein to be healthy. If you decide that you don't want to eat protein that comes from animals, you can get protein from vegetables, beans, and nuts. However, eating vegetable protein alone means you need to eat a wide variety of protein-rich vegetables to make sure you are getting all the nutrition you need so the protein can do the job. Okay, that is over-simplified but it is the best I can do with my own knowledge. I just wanted you to get a hint into this critical part of healthy nutrition.

If you decide to read more about protein, that would be great. However, you could just make sure to include lean protein in your diet. I like to think of protein as a way to nurture my body. I think of it the same as putting gas in my car; I can't move forward without it.

For me, in addition to eating lean meats, eating a wide variety of vegetable sources of protein seems to help me to feel better. It also gives me fiber and other nutrients. I generally eat a little protein at every meal. At the end of most days, I have eaten dairy, meat, vegetable, seeds, nuts, and often eggs. I consider the size of a deck of cards as a good serving size for a piece of meat. I generally assume that if the lean meat is about the size of a deck of cards it is around 200 calories. It is important to be aware of calories without compulsively counting them. I do not care that my calorie count is not exact as long as I am healthy and moving toward that average size body.

Fats (unsaturated, saturated, trans)

Simply put, fat is a part of many foods and your body needs fat to function. Vegetables and fruits have almost no fats. Foods like meats, nuts, oils, butter, milk, cheese have fat. Not all fats are the same. There are unsaturated fats, saturated fats, and trans fats and others. Fats fuel the body and help with vitamin absorption.

Unsaturated fats are generally in plant foods and fish. The best of these are olive oil, canola oil, peanut oil, albacore tuna, and salmon. Some fish have minor amounts of saturated fat as well. Saturated fats are in animal products, meats, butter, cheese, and whole milk. They are also in palm and coconut oils. Saturated fats are not so good for you in that they can have a negative impact on cholesterol. Trans fats are in any product where the ingredients listed on the label say hydrogenated or partially hydrogenated oils. This is bad. Trans fats cause serious health problems. I encourage you to read more about fats. The book that I mentioned earlier was extremely helpful, *Low-Fat Lies High-Fat Frauds and the Healthiest Diet in the World* by Kevin Vigilante, MD, MPH, and Mary Flynn, PhD. (LifeLine Press, A Regnery Publishing Co., 1999). This book changed my food choices forever and provides much more than just information about fats.

For me, I try to stick to olive oil, canola oil, occasional peanut oil, and real butter. Generally, using canola oil, limiting my butter, and trying to be creative with olive oil, makes it easy for me to enjoy what I eat. I understand that there are saturated fats in the meats I eat but I try to eat lean meats, rarely eat beef, and remember that moderation is important.

One reason I gave up dieting and decided to live with my obesity was that I realized I did not know enough about nutrition. Giving up did not work. Using MicroSteps helped me learn to accept that I am not an expert in nutrition and will never know it all but I can educate myself so that I have control over how I fuel my body.

Carbohydrates (complex, simple)

There are two types of carbohydrates. Simple carbohydrates are basically sugar. You find it in candy and cake. Foods like fruits and whole milk have simple carbohydrates as well, but are healthier because of their vitamins, fiber, and other nutrients. Complex carbohydrates include whole grains, vegetables, oatmeal, and whole grain breads. They are not all equal because some are refined. Refining removes some of the nutrients and fibers. Unrefined grains are richer in fiber, which helps your digestive system work. Carbohydrates have a big impact on your blood sugar level. Eating complex carbohydrates will help you avoid hunger longer and be less likely to cause a spike in your blood sugar level.

There is so much more to know; however, this is a beginning and the goal here is to get you to develop an interest in doing your own research and reading. If you are struggling with hunger issues, increasing your knowledge of proteins, carbohydrates, and fats may help you conquer this problem. You do not need to be an expert in nutrition to figure out what you need to know to take care of your own personal food challenges.

We are all a little different. If I eat simple carbohydrates for breakfast, I will end up feeling hungry by 10AM and then snacking to try to fix the problem. For me, I have to eat protein with complex carbohydrates to make sure I am not fighting hunger the rest of the day. An example would be a hardboiled egg and a piece of whole grain wheat toast with a tablespoon of peanut butter. This will get me through at least four hours. If I eat a doughnut for breakfast at 8AM, I will be starving an hour later and eating everything in sight.

The idea here is to get a little knowledge. Use it. If you still have questions, get some more knowledge. Do that until you have enough knowledge to take care of your body. Use the knowledge to help you develop healthy Habits, Routines, Rituals, and Traditions in MicroSteps.

Reading the Ingredients on the Food Label

Okay, so I am not an expert at this either. You do not need to be an expert to know enough to keep your food intake healthy. Here is what I believe to be true. The ingredients listed are in order of the most to the least amounts in the package. For example, if sodium and fructose are the first two things on the ingredient list, I know I am buying a product with a lot of salt and sugar in it. I try to buy products with only few ingredients and those ingredients are words I can pronounce and define. If I do not know what the words mean, I assume I do not know what I am putting into my body. I will occasionally look something up online but most of the time I want to see an easy to read list of ingredients that identify things I actually recognize.

Once I identify the ingredients and consider their order in the list, I ask myself if this something I want to put in my body. Another thing I consider is how often I purchase the product. If it is something I use daily or weekly, then it needs to be healthy. If it is something that I rarely use, I will consider making some occasional allowances for less healthy choices. Of course, there are ingredients I simply do not buy. Trans fats and artificial sweeteners are the main ones in this category. I do not buy anything with the words hydrogenated or partially hydrogenated in the list.

I like to have some quick meal choices that I occasionally use in an emergency. If you use it more than a couple of times a month, it is more of a Habit or Routine. One of these emergency foods is the little combination packages of tuna salad and crackers. I have checked the ingredients and the tuna is healthy enough but not healthy enough for a daily Routine. The crackers have trans fats. Therefore, I just eat the tuna with my own healthy crackers. I toss the crackers that come with the tuna into the trash. I grab a piece of fruit and have myself a quick lunch. I only do this when I have gotten up too late to make a healthy lunch and know there is not going to be time to go out for lunch.

Another example of a quick meal choice is the little frozen cheese and bean burritos. They are about two hundred and forty calories each, have no trans fats; however, they do have some ingredients that I prefer to avoid. They are a processed food with preservatives, use vegetable oil, and have more sodium than I would use if making them from scratch. They help in a crunch when I would be tempted to eat fast food because there's nothing easy in the refrigerator. Again, these are not healthy enough for a daily or even weekly Routine but I find them to be helpful every couple of months. It helps that they are a wonderful balance of satisfying and yet not too delicious. That prevents me from being tempted to eat them too often.

Processed Foods vs. Natural Whole Foods

I define whole natural foods as foods that are fresh from the tree or ground such as fruits and vegetables. It also includes fresh meats. I consider *frozen* vegetables and fruits to be as healthy as fresh vegetables and fruits as long as there are no other ingredients added. Sometimes it is impossible to find the fresh foods you need. Frozen vegetables and fruits last a long time and can come in handy. Some seem to be even better than fresh, such as green peas.

Processed foods are foods that have been changed by adding something or altering them in some way to make them last longer. This includes foods precooked as frozen dinners, packaged meals, or canned food. I also think of fast food as processed food. It is not that I never eat processed foods but that I try to eat mostly whole natural foods. Having said that, when I buy processed foods, I look at a label to see how many ingredients there are, if I know what the ingredients are, and then decide if the product is healthy enough to use. Many processed foods such as tomato sauce, broths, prepared salad dressings, and others are healthy and delicious. You just need to read the labels, especially the ingredients, to make sure they are not loaded with sodium, sugar, or other ingredients you do not want to eat too frequently or as part of your daily Routine.

Portion Control

Portion control can be a challenge in a world of supersizing, extra large servings, and out-of-control appetites. Calorie counting can be helpful in the beginning when you are not sure how much is too much or just what an average size person would eat. In the beginning, I took every opportunity to take a quick peek at average size people's plates to see what they ate and in what portions. I did this at work and at restaurants. I encourage you to do some calorie counting, if you have never done that before. I do not encourage you to do it for life or even for very long; just count calories long enough to educate yourself.

When I began my journey, I did not try to control portions at all. For a long time, I just tried to eat healthy choices. Remember, we do this in MicroSteps. I had planned to address the issue of portion control at some point but the issue addressed me before I could get to it. As I ate healthier whole natural foods, my appetite decreased and my portions became smaller. I would go out to eat, order what would have been a normal size meal in the past, and then end up taking most of it home. I eventually realized that I needed to cook and order less. At first, this scared me. I think subconsciously I was scared that I would end up hungry. After reassuring my inner child that I would take care of her, I was finally able to take a chance on ordering less and cooking less. It is nice; I save money and am still satisfied with my meal.

Fiber (insoluble, soluble)

Fiber is the part of the plants that we cannot digest. It passes through our small intestine and into the colon, keeping the colon healthy. We get fiber in fruits, beans, oats, apples, barley, flax seeds, whole grains, nuts, wheat bran, and vegetables. Two common types of fiber include insoluble fiber and soluble fiber. Insoluble fiber does not dissolve in water and increases the bulk of the stool. Soluble fiber dissolves in water and softens the stools making it easier to pass things through the body. Fiber is good for you.

When I forget to eat fiber (4-5 daily servings of fruits, vegetables, whole grains, nuts), I stop losing weight. My body starts to feel bloated and my stomach does not seem to feel as empty when I am hungry. When I feel like I am losing weight too slowly, based on my daily food intake, I simply have a large salad loaded with fiber. It always works and before I know it, I am losing weight and moving closer to my goal of becoming a healthy, average size person. While there are many high fiber foods I enjoy, I also think of those foods and a way to nurture and make my body healthier. Scientists are always looking for the magic pill that will help us lose weight. For me, that pill is my large salad loaded with healthy vegetables, nuts, and whole grains. Just keep the salad dressing healthy, as well as the ingredients in the salad.

Calories

A calorie is a unit of energy found in all food. We need calories to function. Your physical activity level, gender, and individual body all play a part in how many calories you need to maintain your energy and weight. There are complicated formulas that have something to do with body mass index, height, weight, activity level, and other factors that can help you know how many calories you need to maintain your current weight. They simply confuse me. Not being much of a math person, I have found there is a simple way to get an idea of how much you can eat and lose weight.

I have been doing this simple method for years. I don't remember where I learned it. All I do is to *take my weight and multiply that by my activity level.* The number for the weight is easy; just get on a scale. How do you know your number for activity level? I do not know where the activity numbers come from but for a moderately active woman the number is 12 and 15 for the moderately active male. If you are less active, lower the number by one or two points (women 10, men 13). If you are more active, raise the activity number by one or two points.

For example, a woman weighing 225 pounds who is moderately active (225 x 12 = 2,700) must be eating approximately 2,700 calories to maintain that weight. Once you know what you're eating to maintain your weight, you might need to experiment a little to see what it takes to begin to lose. The idea is that if you eat less than you need to maintain, you will lose.

Again, this works for me but it is not scientific or exact. Playing with these numbers has helped me stay in touch with reality by showing me that I'm overeating. That makes it easier to figure out what type of changes I need to make to continue to lose. I don't spend much time playing with the numbers and don't recommend it. However, it has helped me out from time to time.

For years, I counted every calorie I ate. I lost weight but I gained it all back and more. When counting calories, we need to avoid *all-or-nothing* thinking. I believe that calories do matter. I don't know if all calories are equal but for our journey, I treat them as equal. I think this may be something the experts are still debating.

You need to have an idea of how many calories are in the foods you eat; however, I do not think it is a good idea to count every calorie you eat for the rest of your life. I like to do occasional spot checks to make sure I am not fooling myself about how much I am eating or not eating. Once you have an idea of how many calories are in the foods you regularly eat, you can learn how to estimate the calories in your food choices or meals. You can use the information to make sure you eat only portions that allow your body to get to that healthy, average size. You will learn how to look at that tasty sweet roll and decide it is not worth the calories without knowing exactly how many calories it contains. This is because your knowledge of food reminds you that it is loaded with unhealthy fat, sugar, and white flour. You may not know how to cook it but you know enough to make a better choice for your body.

Hypoglycemic Index

This is all about how our blood sugar responds to certain foods. The Hypoglycemic Index tells us how the food will affect our blood sugar level. It's easy to find lists of the foods and their specific index online.

The proponents of the Hypoglycemic Diets are all a little different in what they tell you to eat or not eat; however, they do have some things in common. They generally tell you to eliminate sugar, white flour, and alcohol. The idea in this is to help you keep your blood sugar level. Diabetics are often on this type of diet and there are other health benefits as well. You are encouraged to eat protein including lean meats, nuts, and dairy products. You are also encouraged to eat whole grains, vegetables, certain fruits, protein, eggs, and plain yogurts.

You may need to experiment a little to notice how your body is reacting to foods such as fruits and vegetables and make sure what you are eating is keeping the blood sugar level. I watch my energy level and pay close attention to how quickly I am getting hungry or craving foods. I expect a healthy meal or snack to hold me comfortably for three to four hours at least.

While I am not suggesting a Hypoglycemic Diet or any other specific diet, I do believe we can learn some things from studying this approach. When I get hungry and want a snack, I remember that if I go for white flour or sugar products my blood sugar will spike then fall, and I will end up tired and hungrier. Since I want to keep my blood sugar level, I will go for whole grain crackers with string cheese or a Kashi bar (whole grains, nuts, and fruit). This gives me the quick energy that will last for a while. For me, protein with complex carbohydrates prevents a spike in blood sugar level and provides a more balanced energy.

If I were to eat a candy bar, I would get a burst of energy and then be dropped like a hot potato. I would end up tired and probably overeating later to try to fix my energy. If you struggle with feeling hungry and wanting to snack, you might want to do some reading on Hypoglycemic Diets and learn which foods are more likely to help keep the blood sugar level.

There is a lot more information about this approach to eating that you can read if you are interested. The books on the subject are endless. For myself, I like to take the parts of the theory that help me out and keep my approach to eating less restricted. Talk to you doctor if you have medical issues related to blood sugar or other health issues.

Fats + Sugars = Palatable

In his book, *The End of Overeating: Taking Control of the Insatiable American Appetite* (Rodale, 2009) author David A. Kessler, MD, discusses the idea that one of the issues related to cravings is that some foods are more palatable than others are. When you combine fats and sugars, he states, the food result is so tasty and palatable that is becomes almost impossible to resist. I believe him. I have experimented a bit with this. If you are struggling with cravings related to sweets, you might want to read his book.

I have not completely given up fats and sugars (desserts) but, as a Routine, I almost never bring them home. If I have a craving for something, I find that it is better to go ahead and have a small serving than to try to resist, think about it for hours, eat everything else in sight, and eventually end up eating more than I would have eaten originally had I not tried to resist. Fortunately, I find eating healthy foods before having an occasional dessert generally inhibits my appetite enough that I do not binge on desserts. It does not work for me to say absolutely "no" to sweets. Remember, this entire process started with my giving up dieting and eating everything I wanted. When I make something completely off limits, my rebellion kicks in and I end up eating badly.

I confess the power of the *palatable* dessert is so strong that it is hard to stop with one serving. It is almost impossible for me to see a doughnut, sweet roll, brownie, or pecan pie and not eat more than one. The only thing that seems to help is to not bring them home and always eat a healthy meal before allowing myself such a treat. Even then, I may struggle for a few days afterward to get back to my healthy eating. When that happens, I specifically rely on established healthy Habits and Routines to keep me on my journey to healthy HRRTs.

Be the Expert You Need to Consult

While you have the above information, it is not enough. I encourage you to continue to educate yourself about nutrition and cooking. There is no shortcut. Knowledge is power and you have to read or do something intentional to increase knowledge. In addition, the field of food and nutrition is constantly growing and changing. We will never know it all and must continue to increase our knowledge to stay up to date.

I encourage you to read from several authors. Do not rely on one study that you heard about on the news. Consider the source of the study. Who will be making money if you buy the product? Find sources that seem to be objective and genuinely interested in teaching you about nutrition. Ask if the author is trying to sell you a product. Question! Think! Ask! Learn! Be the expert you need so that you may depend on yourself to guide your eating and nutrition. Yes, this is hard work and it is time consuming. I believe my life depends on my willingness to make the effort to be educated about nutrition. Education is not only about getting a college degree. Education is about what you put in your head. I want my head filled with knowledge that will give me the power to maintain a healthy, average size body.

Examples of My Lifestyle HRRTs

Everyone's Habits, Routines, Rituals, and Traditions will be different and based on each person's individual likes, dislikes, daily schedule, and unique life situations. As to be expected, our personal HRRTs are subject to change. They change as we achieve more awareness and more knowledge. They also change as our lives naturally evolve with new relationships, environmental changes, and life situations. By the time you read the examples below, my HRRTs will have evolved. This is what I was doing after losing the first sixty pounds.

Below are some examples of my HRRTs to give you an idea of how this works for me. I did not separate my Habits, Routines, Rituals, and Traditions; it does not matter if you perfectly label each behavior. This list is not intended to be all-inclusive but to give you the idea of how to create healthy HRRTs without being too rigid.

Basic (Daily or Almost Daily)

- I have one-two cups of coffee each morning.
- I eat three meals a day and have a snack around 3PM.
- I eat breakfast before 8AM.
- I take my lunch to work.
- I keep healthy snacks in my desk at work.

Occasional (Two to Three Times a Month)

- I order iced tea and sometimes put sugar in it when eating out.

- I skip breakfast, go to brunch around 11AM, and do not eat again until dinner.
- I eat small amounts of chips, salsa, and order Flan at a Mexican Food Restaurant.

Special (Two to Three Times a Year)

- While at an event or working on a project, I may drink coffee all day.
- I participate in a potluck at work and eat whatever suits me.
- I have chocolate cake and vanilla ice cream on my birthday.
- On the day of the holiday (i.e. Thanksgiving, Passover, Christmas), I eat without worrying about weight management.
- I make brownies for my nieces and nephews and eat two or three of them.

Basic Day's Food Intake on an Ordinary Work Day (when working eight to ten hours a day)

Now, this is not what I eat every day, but it shows you what I might eat on a day when I am working. I eat many other things as well. For example, I often take soup, a wrap, or a salad instead of a sandwich for lunch or go out with a friend. I eat a wide variety of things for dinner but this will give you an idea of an ordinary day when I am busy and just trying to get through the day.

Breakfast: two hard-boiled eggs (one yolk), one piece of whole grain wheat toast with a tablespoon of peanut butter, one to two cups of black coffee (10oz)

Lunch: sandwich with two slices of whole grain wheat bread, one slice Provolone cheese, about 3 oz of lean turkey, lettuce, two tablespoons of honey mustard dressing; two pieces of fruit (one is for snack later in afternoon); a small baggie filled with raw vegetables

Dinner: 6-8 oz grilled chicken breast (or pork chop); large salad with lots of raw vegetables with about 4 tablespoons of Balsamic dressing; 1/2 cup brown rice

Optional snacks during the day: (choose one and only if hungry between meals) 1/4 cup of mixed trail mix (not the kind with candy in it), Kashi granola bar, or fruit

Evening Treat (if needed): orange, grapefruit, or a cup of Kashi Cereal (dry)

Note: Generally, I drink water with my meals, unless I go out to eat and then I may have iced tea.

Some General Guidelines

I do have some general guidelines for my eating. This does not mean I always follow them. It means I hope to follow them; however, if I do break one of my guidelines (not calling them rules), I just move on to the next moment without worrying about it. So far, the slips have been rare.

- No Fast Food
- No Trans Fats
- No Artificial Sweeteners
- No Binge Eating and Feeling Sick Afterward
- No More Than 2 or 3 Sodas a Year (regular, never diet)
- Use Only Olive Oil, Canola Oil and Occasionally Peanut Oil
- Use Only Real Butter (no margarines or artificial fats)
- Avoid Processed Foods
- Try to Eat Whole Grains and Avoid White Flour
- Avoid Sugar Most of the Time
- No Alcohol (my personal choice, actually had a margarita twice last year)
- Stop Eating When Stomach Feels Satisfied or Full

Healthy Eating on a Budget

I cannot tell you how many times I have heard someone say that he or she cannot afford to go on a diet or to eat healthy. I have been poor and I have been comfortable. You are right, poor is not fun; being comfortable is definitely better. Of course, poor could mean you have absolutely no money for food and that is an entirely different issue; however, for what we are doing today, let's say you have a small but survivable food budget.

It is much less expensive to do your own cooking from scratch than to buy prepackaged, processed foods, or to go out for fast food. Many healthy foods are within most people's budgets. Foods such as beans, brown rice, fresh vegetables, and fresh fruits are less expensive and healthier than processed and fast foods. It is less expensive to buy a whole chicken or turkey than to buy the parts individually or to buy the sandwich meats. Whole grain pastas can go a long ways on a budget.

Cooking in large portions may also help. It is not that expensive to make a huge pot of healthy vegetable soup or chili and have many meals out of it. Cook a whole turkey and make the most of all the parts, including some turkey soup with the leftovers. Pick up a supersize package of chicken legs and cook them all. I love to do this and freeze them in baggies with two or three in an individual serving baggie. Catch the large bags of prepared salad when they are almost out of date and on sale; buy them and use them that night. Throw some grilled chicken breast on them and call it a healthy dinner for the whole family.

If you are on a budget, it might help to give yourself more time in the grocery store. Walk slowly down the aisles and think creatively as you shop for less expensive items. There are always items on sale. Consider using coupons.

It helps to have some knowledge of cooking so that you can come up with ideas as you see what is on sale. Try to be flexible. Instead of insisting that you make pot roast for dinner and then getting frustrated because it is too expensive, consider switching to whatever is on sale that week. There are even shows on the Food Network that teach preparing meals on a budget.

I understand. It frustrates me too when I have just gotten used to taking peaches for my lunches and then they are no longer on the shelf. This is because we are creatures of Habit. We develop a comfort with what we eat regularly. Do not allow such minor discomforts to throw you off track. The season changes and so does what is available in the stores. Go with the seasons and you will find less expensive items, especially produce.

Cook or Eat Out?

There are a couple of absolutes. First, we must eat to survive. Second, either we eat what we prepare or we eat what others prepare.

How do we determine where to eat? One of the few things in life we can truly control is what we put in our mouths and yet we find eating to be one of the most difficult things to control. There is no right answer to the question: Do I cook for myself or do I eat out? Most people do some combination of the two.

The first decision is to determine where the bulk of your eating will occur. One does not have to eat all three meals and all snacks in the same place. One could eat lunch out daily and still be eating the bulk of one's meals at home. Try not to think in terms of all-or-nothing. It is likely that many factors play a part in the decision. These include, where you live, what you do with your time, your stage of life, your family situation, and your budget.

For those who like to eat out, remember, not all restaurants are equal. One thing for sure about eating out is that unless you are a chef, you probably do not know exactly what is in a dish. If you live in a large city, you have many choices from fine dining to the cheap, unhealthy dives. For those who live in smaller towns, you may not even have a fine restaurant; your best choices may be chain restaurants that serve foods not any healthier than fast foods.

The issues when eating out are different if you are eating out daily or if you are only eating out a few times a month. For those who eat most of their meals at home, eating out is more of a special event or occasional eating experience. That does not mean you need to reward yourself with food, overeat, or go completely overboard with your choices. It does mean that whatever you eat is not part of your regular food intake. For example, I allow iced tea with sugar when I eat out. I eat out around once a week. That means that on a daily basis I am not having iced tea with sugar but am having it occasionally.

I have fewer concerns about eating extra sugar once a week than I do if it becomes a daily Habit or Routine. It is important to remember that white flour, butter, sugar, and such are less healthy choices. I try to eat my best in moderation and without being rigid. For example, I would not buy fresh French Rolls and bring them home each week; however, I do occasionally have a French Roll in a restaurant when I eat out. If I were a person who ate out daily, then I would not have the French Rolls on a daily basis when eating out.

If you are eating out daily, try to eat foods that are natural, fresh, not processed, lower in fats, and have less salt and sugar. Most menus include salads, lean meats, vegetables, and other such items. Remember, if this is your daily Habit or Routine, it is not a special or occasional event. Your food choices on a daily basis have an enormous impact on your health and size. If you eat out daily, you need to consider that before ordering your meal.

For those of us who like to cook for ourselves, there are some similar issues to consider. At least when you eat at home, you know what you are eating. However, that brings us to the question: Can you cook? Can you cook well enough, with enough variety to enjoy what you cook, and prevent those trips to fast food for variety? On the other hand, perhaps you are a great cook and love to cook heavy fattening meals with fabulous desserts. Either way you need to remember that your daily food choices have an enormous impact on your health and body size.

Perhaps you could consider making healthy meals most days and then totally enjoy your cooking creativity to the max once a month, for a special meal with friends or family. There needs to be a difference between your daily cooking and your special event extravaganzas. Daily cooking Habits and Routines needs to be healthy, interesting, tasty, and nutritional.

One thing for sure is that when you cook at home you know what is going into your body. That does give you more power and control over your physical health, as long as you are preparing healthy meals.

Tips for Being Prepared at Home

Almost every weekend, I make some good healthy food to freeze and eat later. This could be a huge pot of Tortilla Soup (Bonus Chapter for recipe) or 6-12 grilled boneless skinless chicken breasts. I keep leftovers in the freezer in individual serving portions. I also prep my favorite raw vegetables and fruits on the weekend and keep them in the refrigerator ready to eat at a moment's notice. (Hint: Wash vegetables, wrap them in a damp paper towel, put them in a baggie, squeeze out most of the air, and refrigerate. They last much longer.)

I like to have some basic favorites in the freezer and refrigerator to use when I am tired, hungry, and willing to eat almost anything (i.e. fast food). I prefer not to eat the frozen dinners from the markets because they are not as good as mine, tend to have too much sodium, and a lot of stuff in the ingredients that I do not understand. My daily foods are simple, basic, delicious, and not processed.

You may ask, "After you freeze them, are they as good as the day they were cooked?" That is a fair question. Some are just as good after being frozen, some are better (like rice), and some are not quite as good. What I can tell you is that they are healthier and generally tastier than fast food or processed frozen dinners. They are easier and faster than cooking from scratch every night after work. They are keeping me healthy and getting me to that healthy, average size body. You figure it out for yourself, but it works for me.

Freezing Food for Later

Freezing the foods is not the challenge. Figuring out how to reheat them is not always easy. If you just throw it in the microwave, you may end up with a mess. When reheating in the microwave, reheated foods can end up uneatable, such as rolls that you cannot even bite. I have a few techniques that work for me and I want to share them with you.

> *Defrost in Refrigerator then Reheat on Stovetop or Microwave:* This technique will work for any type of soups, beans, and most meats. You need to plan ahead with this technique. Put the frozen container in the refrigerator the night before and then reheat the defrosted food in a pan the next morning. Once I defrost a frozen dish, I make sure I eat it the same day or toss it out.

> *Remove from Plastic or Baggie, Put in Glass Dish, then Microwave with a Paper Towel or Paper Plate Covering:* I like to use this technique with my special tortilla soup, stews, marinara sauces, chili, taco meat, chicken legs, black-eyed peas, beans, and rice. When I am ready

to use one of the above dishes, I just remove it from the freezer. If it is in a plastic container, I turn it upside down and run warm water on it for about five seconds. I pop the frozen soup out of the container and put it into a glass bowl. I cover with a paper plate to prevent the microwave from getting dirty, and reheat it in the microwave. If your microwave has a setting for sensory cooking, that is all the better.

Remove the Food from the Container, Put it in Non Stick Skillet with a Tablespoon of Water, Put on a Lid and Reheat on Very Low Temp: This works well with boneless skinless chicken breasts, boneless pork loin chops, meat loaf, meatballs, and leftover turkey. The water will either disappear or turn into a little bit of gravy. It is tasty and easy. You could even use a broth instead of water. If the meat needs to be crisp, take the lid off and just sear it a bit. It works well and I think better than using the microwave to reheat meat.

Eat Frozen or Just Slightly Defrosted: I use this technique with things such as fresh strawberries, grapes, bananas, brownies, candy, nuts, and fresh homemade cranberry sauce. There are no tricks to this. Just take it out of the freezer for a few minutes and enjoy.

Wrap in Damp Paper Towel before Reheating in Microwave: I use this technique for rolls, tortillas, and other bread products. It prevents them from getting hard or rubbery. The trick is to reheat on a low power and for only a few seconds. You can always add time but if you overdo it, your bread becomes hard. Of course, you can also reheat breads in the oven or tortillas on the stovetop.

Let the food come to room temperature before freezing: I have discovered that most foods reheat better if you allow them to come to room temperature before freezing. I think this is because you end up with less steam and condensation. For example, when I've frozen the rice while it is still warm, it is sticky and mushy when reheated, whereas, when I wait until it is cold before putting it into the freezer, it reheats all fluffy and better than ever.

Just remember, when reheating *less is more.* Use lower heat, lower power sittings, and shorter time. You can always add more time and continue to reheat but if your power sitting is too high or you reheat for too long, you will end up with burned or rubbery food. What can I say? MicroSteps even work here! Experiment and figure out what works for you and enjoy your food.

Cooking for One

Okay, I have done this for years. Here is the secret. Other than making breakfast or preparing a lunch to take to work, I do not cook for one. I cook for ten. After cooking, I eat a normal size meal, divide the leftovers into individual servings and freeze or put them in the refrigerator. It is rare that I just cook one serving. When you cook for ten, you only need to cook every few days or weeks.

I will set aside a Saturday or Sunday and cook two or three things for freezing. This could be a pork loin roast, a large pot of chili, my favorite tortilla soup, or a dozen grilled chicken breasts. I do best if I have a variety of foods, all in individual servings, waiting for me after a long day at work. It is like coming home to a fine restaurant and being able to choose from the menu. It is simple; I do not cook for one unless I am making breakfast or a sandwich for lunch.

Stocking the Cupboard

There are some basics that I always have in my kitchen. Of course, my food choices are unique to my likes and dislikes. Since each of us is different, it makes no sense for you to think of this as your grocery list but here is what I like to keep on hand.

As a rule, I have plenty of fresh fruits and vegetables at all times, most of which are in the refrigerator. I always have eggs, butter, non-fat yogurts, some cheeses, healthy salad dressings, bags of salads, and waters in my refrigerator. I keep my freezer stocked with lean meats, individual portions of dishes I have cooked, nuts, frozen fruits and vegetables, and my favorite whole grain breads (yes in the freezer).

In the cupboard, I keep a lot of chicken and beef stock, tomato paste, canned tomatoes, cans of tuna, cans of beans, whole grain pastas, mild green chilies, and my favorite spices on hand at all times. My three favorite spices are kosher salt, lemon pepper, and garlic powder. I also like cilantro, dill weed, basil, thyme, rosemary, parsley, cumin, oregano, cinnamon, chili powder, bay leaves, poultry seasoning, and many others. To top it off, I have a lemon tree and an herb garden in my back yard. I keep limes, onions, fresh garlic, carrots, red bell peppers, toma-toes, and celery on hand as well.

I do not buy many snack foods. Not all snacks are equal. It helps me to understand that a piece of fruit will give quick energy but will not be with me as long as the mixture of nuts and fruits in the trail mix. I always have trail mix (not the kind with candy in it) and Kashi Bars at home. Remember, if you do not buy it, you will not eat it; however, you will eat something. That is good news and bad news. Do not bring home junk foods. Do bring home fresh vegetables and fruits. It is okay to toss out foods that have old dates or gone bad because you did not eat them. Just buy it; you will eventually learn to cook and eat it. I always have fresh garlic in the house; sometimes I use it. If I end up throwing it out, it does not matter. When I use it, it helps make the meal more delicious.

Making the Best Use of the Food Network

You do not need to be a gourmet chef to make use of the Food Network. You do not have to use the exact recipes demon-strated by the chefs on the various shows. It has been fun for me to learn some of the cooking techniques. I apply the skills to my own tastes, using the ingredients I like. I have also learned things about freezing foods, choosing the freshest fruits and vegetables, how to cook and store vegetables, and some fun ideas for products to buy that make cooking and food prep eas-ier. For example, I purchased a garlic press and that has made mincing garlic so easy that I use garlic more frequently. I have learned endless ways to use fresh herbs and that has helped me enjoy my own cooking more. For me, the more I enjoy my own cooking the more likely I am to eat healthy meals.

Taking Charge

There are hundreds of books out there that will tell you how to eat, lose weight, gain weight, be healthy, or otherwise take care of your body. We read the books and put them down; in doing so, we put the knowledge back on the bookshelf with the book. We do not make the knowledge our own. I am not going to tell you exactly how to eat to get that healthy, average size body. I am telling you that you must take responsibility for what goes in your mouth, if you want to control your weight.

What do I mean by taking responsibility for what goes in your mouth? You must intimately understand the basic food groups in order to be a healthy, average size. You need to have a general idea of how the food is prepared, how much to eat, and how often you need to eat so that you can maintain a healthy, average size body. It is important to know how fats affect your health and to understand the effect of white flour and sugar on your appetite and energy. You must have an educated opinion about how to maintain your body. That does not mean that you have to be a nutritionist or dietitian. You just need to be as informed as those folks who do eat healthy and consequently maintain a healthy, average size body.

One author and one book cannot do this for you. Just like one teacher did not give you your entire kindergarten through high school or college education. If you only watch one news channel, you get only one perspective of the world events. If you only shop at one store for clothing, your styles will be limited. If you only read one cookbook, you will cook only one style of food. Take the challenge, get out there, and research. I do not take any medications until I have read about them and their possible side effects. I like to think of food as being as powerful as any drug. I need to know about food and nutrition because when I overdosed on food, I ended up 315 pounds. That did not work for me!

Bonus Tips

- I always have water on my desk when I am at work.

- I intentionally have a snack in the afternoon, if I know dinner will be late.

- I keep my kitchen, including my refrigerator, clean to make it easier to cook a healthy meal.

- I try to make the food I prepare at home as delicious as or better than what I could buy in a standard fast food or chain restaurant.

- I eat slowly to give my stomach a chance to let me know when it is full; I stop eating when I feel full.

- When I have eaten enough food for an average meal (or healthy small snack), I stop eating whether I feel full or not. I cannot always trust my brain to tell my stomach to inform me that I am full.

CHAPTER 6

Show Me the Evidence

HOW'S IT GOING? By now, you have learned how to pick small easy-to-change Habits, Routines, Rituals, or Traditions and how to make changes in MicroSteps. As mentioned before, Habits are the easiest to change; Routines more difficult, Rituals even more difficult, and Traditions much more deeply imbedded in our hearts. Just something to keep in mind as your journey continues.

Evidence of Progress

The first sign that you are making progress is that some of your HRRTs have changed. I would encourage you to make a list of just how your HRRTs have changed. It is easy to forget where we have been once we are in a new place. If fact, that is how this book started. I began taking some notes because I needed to keep track of my own progress and of what I was learning. This book is the result of my notes. Remember, progress is not about leaps and bounds; it is like the turtle's race in MicroSteps.

In addition to observing how your HRRTs are changing, there are some other simple ways to identify that you are making progress in your journey to a healthy, average size body. You might consider having a physical so that you can see if your blood pressure, cholesterol, or other medical problems have improved. Of course, you can always take out a tape measure or get on the scale to see the evidence of weight loss. Have you been shopping for clothes? Are you buying smaller sizes? Are you spending more on clothes every few months because your old clothes are too big? Perhaps, you are spending less on food, finding it easier to fit into chairs, or have increased energy. These are the easiest signs of progress to spot, but there are others.

Have you noticed fewer unhealthy cravings? Are you finding it easier to say, "No" to unhealthy foods? When you do eat cake, do you find that you no longer go on a dessert binge for days afterward? Are you going out more often socially instead of isolating because of embarrassment about the way you look? Have you noticed that you can walk and breathe at the same time? Can you begin to feel your bones when you touch your face, waist, or hips? Are you obsessing less about foods that are not healthy for you? Have you been avoiding fast food? Maybe you have not even noticed. Remember to keep that self-observation going! It will see you through.

The idea is to look for clues that you are making progress. Of course, you want to see the scale numbers go down but that is not the only way to measure progress. The scale may move down so slowly that you feel you will never get to an average size. It is important to look for other signs of progress so that discouragement does not take over. It took me a long time of working on my HRRTs before the weight began to drop off. Then, because I was only losing two to four pounds a month, I could have missed my progress without careful observation. That's okay! I have now lost over eighty pounds and am still losing. By the time you read this, I will have lost more, at a snail's pace, and in MicroSteps. I like to think that going slowly allows my skin to shrink back into place a little. Maybe not, but I like to think that anyway.

Checking Up on Your Progress

While you are not on a diet, you do need to do some intentional eating and food management to reach your healthy, average size. This will both help you lose weight and show you just how far you have come in your journey. One thing I do, on random days, about every six weeks or so is count the calories from the day before. I always do this as an afterthought. I never plan it, like a random drug test. This is important because I believe calories do matter and I do not want to fool myself about how much I am eating.

It is also a good idea to check your general diet occasionally to make sure it is healthy and balanced. Do this about once a month and take the time to recall what you are eating over a week. This is not about calories but about the balance of protein, fats, sugars, carbohydrates (simple and complex), dairy, breads, grains, nuts, and everything else you are eating. Check out www.choosemyplate.com, recommended by the USDA, or use your favorite nutritionist as a resource.

It is also important to check and see how you are doing with complex carbohydrates. Are you eating fresh fruits and vegetables? Are all of your carbohydrates made of white flour and sugar? This could be a problem. I have noticed over the years that when I eat fruits, vegetables, and whole grains my body works better. I feel better, have more energy, and lose weight more regularly. I cannot say why, but I know it works.

Check to see how often you are eating fresh healthy whole foods versus how often you are resorting to processed or fast foods. Become aware that many places, not only the drive-through restaurants, have processed or fast food. You can find fast and processed foods in many inexpensive restaurants as well as in the freezer section of the grocery store. Be aware!

Enjoy fully each pound you lose. I get on the scales every morning to check my progress. To prevent overwhelming myself with the idea that I need to lose what seems like a thousand pounds, I focus only on one *decade* at a time (i.e. ten pounds at a time). I like to weigh daily but that may or may not work for you. Remember, you have to deal with the very special individual that is you, so experiment and see what's most comfortable for your unique personality.

Below, to sum this up, is what works for me:

- I think of ten pounds as a *decade* and focus only on losing ten pounds at a time.

- I weigh daily, usually at same time, and on same scale. I actually weigh on the doctor's scale at my office and on my scale at home. They are about two pounds different. I think of the larger weight (the doctor's scale) as the accurate scale, not that it matters. (After I wrote this, I purchased my own doctor's scale and now only weigh at home but more about that later.)

- Whether I gain, lose, or remain the same, I analyze what I ate the previous day and notice how that affected my weight.

- About once a month, I take a tape measure and measure my waist and anything else that strikes me such as thighs or upper arms.

- I keep an Excel spreadsheet of my progress. I weigh, use a tape measure, and note the size clothing I am wearing. I do this every month or every few months.

Issues Identified or Resolved

Have you notice that your coping skills are improving? Are you managing your irritability better? Do you take a walk when you feel anxious, instead of snacking? This journey is all about the self-observation and empowerment you will experience as you learn more about your Habits, Routines, Rituals, and Traditions (HRRTs). No one has perfect mental health. We all have issues that need further attention. It is important to know yourself so that you can attend to the feelings and behaviors related to the negative HRRTs that are preventing you from achieving that healthy, average size body. As you have been considering your own issues, have you identified something you need to work on? If you have, then celebrate! The progress is in the journey, not in being perfect or arriving at some amazing end.

Most of us are not aware that we are using HRRTs to manage our emotions. Everyone has a crisis, an emotional issue, a celebration, and numerous events that create anxiety or stress. By now, you are becoming aware that we react by returning to our HRRTs for comfort in times of crisis, happiness, boredom, stress, and sadness often mindlessly.

Be your own therapist. We all have moments when we are impulsive, compulsive, or obsessive. We hear these words often and yet many people have no idea what they mean or how they influence our food intake. Here is how I define them:

- *Impulsive* is something you do without thinking at all.

- *Compulsive* is something you feel driven to do and not doing it causes anxiety.

- *Obsessive* is thoughts that you cannot get out of your head.

Based on the definitions above, can you find ways in which they influence your eating? How are they linked to your Habits, Routines, Rituals, or Traditions? Think about it for a while and see if you can find a connection.

Perhaps, related to your obsessions or compulsions, are issues with other people. Maybe they are even connected to memories from your childhood. Look at the following chart to see if you are in a cycle of eating badly which could be connected to your emotions or relationships in some way. Remember, awareness is progress. Are you more aware these days?

Breaking the Cycle of Eating Badly

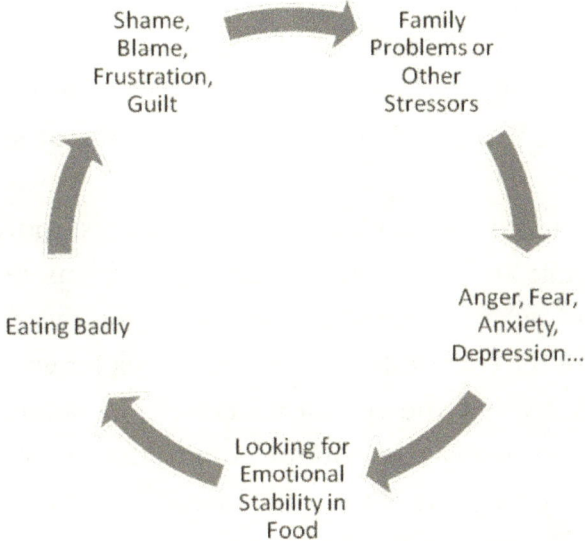

Shame, Blame, Frustration, Guilt

Family Problems or Other Stressors

Anger, Fear, Anxiety, Depression...

Looking for Emotional Stability in Food

Eating Badly

In the above chart, you can see an example of how life stressors and feelings can get us into trouble with food. In this example, you might begin with a family problem or other life stressor. This leads to feelings of anxiety, depression, anger, fear, or some other emotional upset. Not knowing what to do, you begin to look for comfort and emotional stability in food. You give in and eat badly. Suddenly, instead of being upset about the original problem, you are experiencing shame, guilt, frustration with yourself, and blaming yourself for being overweight. This leads you to being irritable and unavailable emotionally to family and friends. The cycle repeats.

The original problems are still there with the family or friends but now you have added your irritability and self-blame to the mix. You do not know what to do with your feelings and so you look to food for comfort and stability, continuing the cycle of eating badly.

To break the cycle you need to change one of the parts. Of course, it would be great if you just stopped turning to food for comfort. You could also change any of the other pieces of the cycle.

If you do slip and eat badly for comfort, just move on without the guilt and shame that increases your emotional upset. You could get into counseling with your family member and try to solve the core problem. You could look for emotional stability in individual therapy for yourself, or by taking a walk, or journaling, or many other options rather than eating. The idea is to identify the parts of the cycle that reflect your HRRTs and begin in MicroSteps to change one small piece of the cycle. One change will lead to another until you are no longer eating badly when upset.

Perhaps you have already changed some of the above cycle and did not realize it until now. As you are trying to find evidence of progress, remember that awareness is progress. Identifying a next MicroStep is progress. Of course, seeing the weight go down is a goal but looking for small changes will give you the encouragement you need to continue to take MicroSteps toward that healthy, average size body.

Traditions in Your Life

When it comes to changing major family Traditions such as holidays, birthday celebrations, weddings, or funerals, pick your battles. You can succeed in this journey without expecting your entire extended family to change the family traditions. Embedded deeply into our hearts, Traditions bind us to our family history, connecting us to each other and to our beliefs. Do not panic when the holidays come around. As you develop a taste for healthy foods, get used to eating average size portions, and learn to manage your emotions, the holiday Traditions will become easier.

Since beginning this journey, I have discovered that my *wants* have changed. My family still has massive amounts of holiday foods and most of it loaded with unhealthy ingredients. I do not reach for it as I did in the past. Now, do not get me wrong, I still eat that piece of pecan pie! But my newly birthed *wants* cause me to enjoy the salad, vegetables, and lean meats that were always served with the meal. I suppose I simply did not notice the healthy stuff before because my personal HRRTs were driving my cravings for the desserts and fattening casseroles.

Keep in mind, knowledge is power. Awareness is an outcome of knowledge. Even if you absorbed everything you have read thus far, you will still need to work on increasing your knowledge of your own feelings, desires, wants, needs, and cravings in order to become fully aware of the unhealthy Habits, Routines, Rituals, and Traditions that are keeping you overweight. Use the steps below to help you with the process and take as long as you need to get through these steps. You will see that we have been doing these steps all along.

1. Identify emotional or behavioral issues that may be preventing you from being ready to begin this journey.

2. Discover your normal eating pattern.

3. Relax. Stop the fad and rollercoaster diets. Eat whatever you want, as you allow yourself to heal from restrictive dieting followed by the *making up eating*. You know, the pizza, dessert, and junk food binges that you go on because certain foods were *off limit* on diets.

4. Each day promise yourself that you may eat whatever you want to eat. This important step will help to heal the emotional damage done by all of those diets and failed attempts at weight loss. (Exception: If you have a medical condition that limits certain foods, follow your doctor's instructions.)

5. Begin to identify your comfort zones. I am talking about those Habits, Routines, Rituals, and Traditions (HRRTs) that, although comforting, are getting you into trouble with food.

6. Select one Habit that, once changed, will help you achieve your goal of ending your war with food.

7. Try to identify a tiny part or MicroStep of that Habit that will be easy to change and give you a feeling of success quickly (two scoops of ice cream after dinner instead of three, four packets of sugar in your tea instead of five).

Taking it One Meal at a Time

Following is a cut from my Self-Observation Journal, written on October 9, 2009, as I was evaluating my own eating Habits, Routines, Rituals, and Traditions:

I started this process by trying to create the Habit of eating a healthy breakfast, and not worrying about the other meals. It was easier with breakfast because I enjoy having the same thing for breakfast daily. Lunches and dinners seem more complicated because I do not eat the same thing for every meal.

Breakfast: Most of the time I enjoy two scrambled eggs and a slice of wheat toast for breakfast with coffee. Occasionally, when I go out or on a weekend, I will make something else. This seems to be working and is Habit/Routine that I will keep for now.

Lunch: When I am working, I generally take my lunch. Most of the time, I take a sandwich, two pieces of fruit, some raw vegetables, and maybe a yogurt or nuts for a snack in the late afternoon. At work, lunches are scheduled and I eat around noon each day. Sometimes I am tired of sandwiches and bring soup for lunch.

Weekends: I tend to eat both breakfast and lunch later in the day. Sometimes I will eat a full meal for lunch and then skip dinner or have a snack. Other times, I skip lunch and eat a larger earlier dinner. I have not resolved my weekend lunch issues at this time and need to continue to look for healthy weekend lunch Habits.

Dinner: I often eat too much dinner. When I was a child, dinner was the main meal of the day and it was always meat, potatoes, gravy, bread, and maybe a vegetable (often corn). We did not eat many vegetables or salads in my family growing up. While my choices are generally much healthier nowadays, I am still eating too large portions and eating too late in the evening.

While I am proud to say that I no longer eat fast food for either dinner or lunch, making dinner a main meal of the day is a Habit/Routine I am working to change. It is one of the most difficult because with that main meal comes a feeling of relaxing, letting go of the stress of the day, and settling into a good book or some television. The idea is to consider how to get those needs met without the Habit/Routine of making dinner a main meal.

Thoughts to Support Healthier Eating

Have you noticed a difference in the way you are handling the day-to-day challenges of life? We all approach problem solving or change in our own special manner. For example, some people are very orderly and organized maybe even a little rigid in their Habits, Routines, Rituals, and Traditions. Others are more laid back and do not hold onto such things so tightly. You must understand your own style and ways in order to become comfortable with changes.

My own style includes a preference for eating things that look like those served in a fine restaurant. For example, I will place a strawberry and slice of orange on the side of my place at dinner. It suggests that I care and makes me feel more nurtured. Have you become more aware of your own style?

Awareness is so powerful. Make a note of where you are becoming more aware. As a new Habit, I was buying healthy things to take to work for lunches (fruits, Kashi Bars, freshly sliced turkey from the deli, yogurts) and only eating them for lunches when I went to work. It finally dawned on me that these healthy foods could also work at any time, any day, anywhere, and I did not have to go to work to eat them. I realized I had been doing that for years. Upon reflection, I remember my mother telling me as a child to leave certain foods alone because they were for school lunches. I had never thought about it before and therefore developed the Habit of not eating the lunch foods at any place other than work.

Old HRRTs are automatic and sometimes easier to break than we realize. This one was actually easy to break, as soon as I became aware of what I had been doing. It helped me to be able to eat these easy, healthy foods any time. You see, I had been struggling with needing an occasional small snack and was not allowing myself to eat the obvious. The answers were right in front of me all the time and I could not see them. Don't let small insights slip past you. Keep a list. Then look at it occasionally so that you remember you have made progress.

Entertain Your Taste Buds

On February 21, 2010, I noticed that I was craving something but could not identify what I wanted to eat. I was struggling again, to my surprise, with a desire for fast food and sugary sweets. I finally stopped wondering if my hormones were out of whack and asked myself why I no longer wanted to eat the healthy foods I had been eating. What was wrong with my lovely new Routine? Eventually, I realized that I had gotten bored eating the same tortilla soup and turkey sandwiches day after day. I had gotten lazy with my cooking and my taste buds were bored. I quickly changed my menu and added some variety, used different spices, mixed things up a little, and the cravings went away. I had not realized that being bored with my meals might cause me to want to return to old HRRTs and thus old comfort foods. What a surprise to discover that boredom could include my taste buds getting bored. Insight! What insights are you noticing? Insights are evidence of progress.

This led me to understand that so much of our eating is unconscious. How many times have you tried to remember what you had for lunch, breakfast, or dinner? I decided to become more conscious of my eating experiences. That is to say, I want to notice the taste, the texture, the colors, and the entire experience. I had been eating while walking around, doing errands, driving, watching television, inputting data into a computer, and socializing. Rarely was I completely paying attention to what I was eating. I wanted to become more aware of my own responses to the meal: Am I satisfied? Do I feel full? Am I eating to manage feelings? Am I eating when I am not hungry? Am I fully enjoying what I am eating or just eating what is there? If this is a challenge for you, you might want to do some reading on *mindful eating*.

Breaking the Ice Cream Habit

I love ice cream. Realizing that I was no longer eating ice cream before bed every night was a time for celebration—evidence of progress. In the past, it was difficult for me to avoid ice cream completely. However, if I allowed ice cream at all, it was difficult to stop with one serving. I wanted to eat it daily. I wanted to eat mountains of it. My love for ice cream threatened to destroy any hopes I had of being able to achieve my goal of having a healthy, average size body, unless I could find a way to control the ice cream binges without having to give up ice cream altogether. Finding my way in this was a true challenge, as I did not intend to terminate my relationship with ice cream totally.

Again, it was time to look at my Habits, Routines, Rituals, and Traditions. It would seem that they were all playing a part in this love affair. I had a Habit of eating ice cream every night before bed. It was part of my nightly Routine, signaling my brain to begin to shut down and prepare for sleep. I had eaten ice cream nightly for so long that it had become a Ritual of comfort and self-nurture. Our family Tradition mandates that we eat ice cream at every birthday party, anytime we eat cake, with most pies, on top of Jell-o, on top of puddings, with cobblers, and underneath chocolate syrup. This was hitting me on every level.

Thank heaven for MicroSteps! The first step was to stop bringing ice cream home on a weekly basis. That meant that I could still buy it for holidays and special events but not keep it around as a staple in my freezer. That did cut down on the binges; however, I missed it terribly. I decided to allow myself to order it when eating out and that helped. By ordering it in public, I have a normal serving, eat it slowly, and continue to enjoy the company of my dinner companion. I make sure never to go to the grocery store right after eating ice cream at a restaurant and that prevents me from buying more.

Another thing that helped was to keep on hand foods that were cold to swallow and sweet but that did not have the power over me like that of ice cream. I discovered frozen fruit, Italian ices, super cold yogurts (not frozen too much like ice cream), and orange juice. These all helped at night while I was beginning a detox from my ice cream addiction. At first, I allowed myself to eat plenty of my substitutes; surprisingly, over time I reduced the portion sizes with minimal effort. I think that is because as I lost weight, my stomach wanted less food.

Did you know that you could take your favorite brand of 100% orange juice and turn it into a delicious frozen fruit (Italian ices style) treat? All you need to do is poor the juice into a casserole dish, the kind that is two inches or so high and rectangle. Stick it in the freezer. About every thirty to forty-five minutes, take a fork and scrape all the sides and bottom. Continue scraping every forty-five minutes to keep it from becoming solid. The scraping is what makes the delicious little ice particles. Once it has frozen into lovely little ice particles, scoop it up, put it into a covered container, and keep it in the freezer. Enjoy it when you have an urge for ice cream. Try the trick with other kinds of juice.

To sum up the ice cream affair: I still enjoy ice cream and usually only have it when I am eating out, often with a drizzle of chocolate syrup. Interestingly, since ending my nightly affair with ice cream, having it only as dessert when eating out, I am experiencing it as a treat instead of feeling guilty for indulging. I actually enjoy it more because the guilt is gone. When I order it, I eat it slowly to make it last. Lately, I have noticed that frequently I don't even think of ordering dessert. My *wants* have changed and so will yours.

One trick I learned during grocery shopping is to substitute a DVD purchase for ice cream and chocolate. I will explain. Whenever I am grocery shopping and began to crave ice cream or chocolate, I stop what I am doing and push my cart over to the DVD rack. I find one I have not seen and buy it. It is wonderful and no more expensive than the ice cream or choco-late would have been! My attention is completely distracted from the ice cream or chocolate. I go home and have a fabulous movie to watch while eating something healthy. It is true. I really do this. It honestly works. The interesting thing is that I have not needed to do it very often. I have probably redirected myself to the DVD purchase system less than twenty times. As eating Habits change, your cravings change. This is good because I do not want to end up with millions of DVDs. What tricks have you learned that are helping you make those Micro-Steps of change? The tricks are part of the progress.

Intentional Grocery Shopping

The first place I shop in the grocery store is the produce sec-tion. I find this is a good way to get my brain thinking about healthier foods. Once I see what produce is fresh and looks good, I have a better idea of what to buy that will complement the produce. This is the opposite of my old way of grocery shopping. In the past, I would randomly walk up and down the aisles picking up whatever struck me. Now, I never go grocery shopping without a list. This helps me focus. I am more likely to keep my shelves stocked with healthy foods and staples if I make a list and *intentionally* grocery shop instead of relying on my impulses. It is also important to keep in mind that the folks who stock those shelves and display items are counting on you to be impulsive.

One day while grocery shopping, I was tempted to stock up on those calorie controlled snacks because I remembered *The Today Show's* nutritionist, Joy Bauer saying it was better to buy those individually wrapped calorie controlled snacks. She said that would help with portion control. I must say, that is not what I had experienced in the past. When I bought a box of low calorie individually wrapped servings of candy, cookies, or ice cream bars, I would eat the entire box the day I brought it home. That approach only works for people who are already in control of their impulsive eating. I do not believe it works for the seriously obese person who is struggling not to eat everything in sight. Since I was learning to think for myself and trust my knowledge, I passed right by those little temptations.

It is better for me to buy a small container of ice cream, one candy bar, or a small package of cookies. That way, if I eat the entire thing, I have only eaten one large portion at one sitting and there is no more in the house. I cannot binge. I have allowed myself to eat something that I was craving and then I can immediately return to my healthy eating Habits/Routines because that is what is in my home. It is over and I have not felt deprived. If it is happening more than once a month, I look at the related HRRTs. I then figure out how to make a small change, in MicroSteps, so that I can manage my cravings in a way that supports my healthy, average size body.

This, as you know by now, is a journey. It is slow and it is in the slowness that you will gain confidence in your ability to succeed. In the small day-to-day successes, you will find your strength and your joy. Look for those small successes. Take my tips, perhaps make a note of your own tips that you might want to share with others, and find joy in the small Micro-Steps of success.

CHAPTER 7

Befriending the Changes and Struggles

AS YOU EXPLORE THE WORLD of your HRRTs, you'll experience a gradually growing awareness of your physical body, relationship to food, social life, increasing knowledge, and yourself. It seems to never end. It is important to notice the small changes in your body. For example, while I was shaving my legs, I noticed that my ankles were thinner and I had to be more careful not to nick myself. This is because my bones were starting to make an appearance as the layers of fat were melting. Bones are bumpier! Who knew? Actually, I noticed this after a rather big nick one morning while I was rushing to get out of the house.

I looked in the mirror and noticed my back seemed to be thinner. This happened one morning when I was trying to figure out why the top I had on suddenly seemed to be showing more cleavage than was within my comfort zone. I rejoiced and decided to alter my comfort zone. I also put on a necklace that I hoped would attract the eye so that my cleavage was not center stage.

Consider this. Your body may still be larger than average but it will be changing nonetheless. Being aware of these small physical changes will help you realize that you are moving slowly toward your goal of being a healthy, average size. It is helpful to understand how your body is responding physically to the changes based on what you are eating. It is also helpful to understand how you are responding emotionally, socially, and mentally to the changes in your body.

I have noticed that my walk has a little of that old bounce to it that it had when I was younger and a bit full of myself. My knees don't hurt so much when I walk; they still hurt some due to arthritis. On the other hand, I simply feel better about my appearance, feel okay in public, and have more energy. It is hard to believe that I walked at all carrying so much extra weight. I can't even lift more than twenty-five pounds without help. I know that because my two cats together weigh about twenty-five pounds and I need help getting their carrier into the vet's office. A delightful energy boom began as soon as I had lost around twenty pounds, and I have noticed that it just gets better and better with each few pounds. It is so exciting that I feel like shouting to the world, "Look at me! I am average again! I feel okay in my own skin!"

I am noticing that these physical and emotional changes contribute to my desire to get out and live more life. I want to go shopping, spend time with friends, catch a movie, take a walk and the irony of it all is that this energy results in increasing my physical, social, mental, and emotional exercise. The more I lose, the better I feel. When I feel better, I move more, which causes me to lose more, which causes me to move more, and I just keep feeling better and better. Now I can live with that cycle!

Without journaling or compulsively counting calories, I try to be aware of what I have eaten from one day to the next. I do this so that I may understand how what I ate yesterday affects today's weight. If I lose a pound, what helped me do that? Not so surprising, I often lose weight after eating a light soup or salad for dinner. I may gain a pound after eating something high in sodium.

If This… Then That

Why are these observations so important? You are eating to support a healthy, average size body. For me, this is new territory. It requires a great deal of self-observation and detailed awareness of how your body reacts to what you are eating. Pay close attention to what is happening to all aspects of your emotional, physical, spiritual, and mental self. Notice "if this… then that" and use that self-observation and knowledge to help move you forward.

Once I learned to observe the changes in my body, I became aware that as little as five pounds seems to make a difference. It becomes obvious in my body shape, my energy, and the way my clothes fit. When you have over a hundred pounds to lose, there is the tendency to dismiss the positive changes achieved by losing two to five pounds.

Learning to identify what triggers weight gain and unwanted eating is critical. Once you know what causes you to want to eat, and how your body responds to what you eat, then you can create MicroSteps to deal with the challenges.

For me, understanding the vulnerability of the five senses has been important in discovering the things that trigger cravings or impulsive eating. The five senses of *seeing, tasting, touching, smelling,* and *hearing* seem to be almost as powerful as the HRRTs. Try to pay close attention to what is happening with your five senses and observe how they connect you to food cravings and impulsive eating.

Actually, I think the five senses drive us to return to the safe old comfortable HRRTs. For example, when I was a preteen, my friends and I loved slumber parties. We always had pizza at these parties. For years, every time I heard the word pizza, smelled pizza, or saw one on television, I would end up ordering pizza from any pizza joint that would deliver. While I have not tried to change my pizza passion, one payoff of the many changes to my Habits, Routines, Rituals, and Traditions, is that I am no longer in love with pizza. This is likely because I have developed a craving for healthy foods. I still like pizza and enjoy it occasionally. I now prefer it to be a healthier version. The fast food type pizza simply no longer controls my emotions or draws me to it as if it were the love of my life.

I have observed that eating healthy food is more satisfying, keeps my blood sugar from extreme changes, and prevents me from impulsively craving unhealthy foods. I try to nurture my body with good food eaten at regular intervals. By eating before I am starving, I no longer have that impulse to grab a greasy pizza, cake, ice cream, pie, cheeseburgers, fries, or ribs. My healthy HRRTs have given me the power to manage my cravings.

Fear of Hunger and Using Portion Control

After losing around thirty pounds, I was getting full much more quickly and it was taking me longer to get hungry again. Amazingly, I had learned to notice the presence or absence of hunger. There is an empty feeling that that happens just before you are hungry and ready to eat. It is nice and I have learned to enjoy it. It just seemed like all of a sudden my stomach would not hold the large portions. What a surprise!

In learning to enjoy a brief moment of hunger, I have lost my fear of feeling hungry. Before I understood how to eat to help manage my blood sugar, I would get hungry and physically shaky as if I were going to faint. I would eat quickly and tell myself that I should not allow myself to become hungry. Now, when I feel hungry I eat a healthy meal, have a Kashi Bar, enjoy some nuts and fruit, or grab some string cheese. It is easy and I do not need to panic because I find myself hungry. That removes a lot of pressure and I eat less because I am not trying to eat to prevent hunger from attacking my body. Hunger is no longer my enemy.

Suddenly, or so it seemed, I was preparing the same portions as always and yet feeling as though I were eating far too much. I knew it would be okay to cut the portion sizes in half and yet I felt a panicky feeling about serving myself less food because, "What if I can't go back for seconds, if I still feel hungry?" A half sandwich was filling me up. Four ounces of meat was as much as I wanted and yet I was still making whole sandwiches and serving myself six or seven ounces of meat. Did this anxiety, related to smaller portions, come from a deeper place? Was this just another Habit that needed my attention? I knew that I had the financial means to make sure I never needed go hungry and yet I felt emotionally that I must eat a certain amount or I might get hungry and not be able to get to food quickly enough.

What a shock it was to discover that I was able to simply eat a bowl of soup for dinner and feel satisfied. That was a major *ah ha* moment! One Habit I worked on was that of being able to feel okay about eating less when less is what fills me up.

For me, there is a danger in waiting until I am too hungry before I eat. When I am too hungry, I tend to eat as if I will starve any second. I overeat and then have regrets. I seem to do better when I eat three meals a day at normal meal times and rarely snack.

As I began noticing that I was satisfied with eating smaller portions, the challenge was then to reduce the amount of food I was eating for lunch and dinner. My MicroSteps had gotten me to the place where I was eating primarily healthy foods. The problem was that I was still eating more food than the healthy, average size body would need. I reassured myself that I could eat less and, if needed, I could go always go back for seconds. Eventually, I just ate less and did not want the seconds. I discovered that I was eating more because of the Habit of loading up the plate. It had not even occurred to me that I could start with small portions and get seconds if I was still hungry or just wanted a little more.

I also noticed that I was eating as if I would *never see that particular food again*. Remember, you can freeze the leftovers or just eat them the next day. I began writing down my favorite recipes so that I could reproduce that favorite vegetable dish, soup, or casserole again. In the past, I had a Habit of just throwing meals and dishes together. Since I am a decent cook, whatever I made was usually good but I could not always reproduce the dishes. Thus, I ended up eating as if I would never have that food again. Writing down my recipes in the computer was not difficult and it made a huge difference in my eating Habits.

Before I began to lose weight, I thought I would need to address all the issues in all my meals, including portion control before my body would lose weight. Amazingly, when I started to lose weight, I had not made any adjustments to portion control for my dinner meals. I was eating healthy foods most of the time but I was still eating far too much for dinner. My body just decided to start losing weight, without waiting for me to take all the MicroSteps needed to eat smaller amounts at dinner.

This was a lovely surprise! My body was changing before I even addressed all the HRRTs that I thought were causing me to be overweight, but I continued to work toward portion control in my dinner meals anyway. The reason is that the less you weigh the fewer calories it takes to maintain that weight. I knew that at some point I would need to eat less to reach and maintain that healthy, average size body. Remember, the goal is not only to lose weight but also to eat to maintain a healthy, average size body.

Monitor the Struggles

It is important to pay attention to the ongoing struggles and conflicts you encounter while establishing healthy Habits, Routines, Rituals, and Traditions. Celebrate that you have become aware of the struggles and conflicts rather than allowing them to pull you back into behaviors that caused you to become overweight in the first place. Keep in mind that changes made slowly, in MicroSteps, gently, and over time, are more likely to stick because they do not create the anxiety that causes you to return to food for comfort.

The day I stepped on the scale and saw that I had lost forty pounds, I was beside myself. It was exciting and I wanted to go shopping, again! I was not yet in mainstream clothing sizes but could see them right around the bend. I was anxious to share my knowledge with others. I felt so much thinner, normal, and fabulous until I looked in the mirror and realized that I was still overweight with about 100 pounds more to lose. Losing forty pounds made me feel so much thinner and yet I was still in plus sizes and extremely large. There was a definite disconnect between how I felt and how I looked. If I were not so aware of my feelings and the process in general, I might have ended up discouraged and returned to my old HRRTs.

I have a passion for cheeseburgers and fries. It is probably my second favorite food. Eggs are my favorite, any style. In the beginning, I found it very difficult to give up cheeseburgers and fries. I finally realized I did not need to make such a sacrifice. I do a lot of my own cooking. Therefore, while I may still have a cheeseburger with fries, I generally make them at home. I either oven-roast the fries or used a small amount of Canola Oil in a skillet. My home cooked cheeseburgers are made of 90/10 lean ground sirloin, or ground turkey, with a limited amount of cheese. They are on a whole grain bun and served with a salad as well as fries.

On rare occasions, I may even go out to a nice restaurant and order a cheeseburger with fries. I am talking about the kind of restaurant where they use real, whole food, no trans fats, and good quality meats. I probably eat a cheeseburger and fries three to four times a year. It is one of my favorite meals.

Warning: Do not try to give up your favorite foods. Instead, find a way to have a healthy version that is flavorful and fulfilling. I find that I actually crave cheeseburgers and fries less often because when I do have them now they are healthy and satisfying. Since I know I can have them at any time, there is no need to panic and have them today.

When eating out it is often difficult to determine the content of the food and the appropriate portion that would support a healthy, average size body. Even though I have been on this journey for a while, it is still a challenge at some restaurants.

Doing my own cooking gives me a sense of power and control over what I am eating, and ultimately over my health. I feel successful when I have cooked a healthy meal and that feeling of success increases my hope for eventually being a healthy, average size person. Doing my own cooking gives me a deeper knowledge of food and what is in the foods at a restaurant. This is powerful knowledge and helps me make healthier choices over the long run. This goes a long way to increasing my self-esteem and my confidence. I believe I can trust myself to take care of my body and my nutritional needs because I have spent the time gaining enough knowledge to do it.

It was difficult to add vegetables to my daily eating. My life did not allow time for all that chewing. Salads take so long to eat and seem to take up an entire lunch break. It was so much easier to eat French fries or a big bowl of macaroni and cheese.

Learning how to cook vegetables helped me immensely in my efforts to keep my food Habits and Routines balanced. You must commit to gaining knowledge. It is okay to learn a little bit at a time and then in MicroSteps put that knowledge into action. I now eat fruits and vegetables on a daily basis. I cannot explain why, but when I eat foods with fiber, such as fruits and vegetables, I seem to lose weight more consistently. I also feel more energized and less bloated.

Grocery shopping can be frustrating because it is not always possible to find quality fresh fruits and vegetables. In the past, when I could not find the fruits or vegetables I had a Habit of eating, I would just give up and go buy something less healthy. I had to learn to be flexible. Again, this happened in MicroSteps.

For example, I decided to start buying a few produce items that were not on my list and just see what I could do with them at home. It took a while, but I finally learned; when I cannot find my first choice, I try something else. Perhaps my first choice is not in season, or is just not fresh that day. I often buy frozen fruits and vegetables; I have learned that some are just as good as fresh. If there are no apples in the store, buy pears. Try something that you have not tried before.

This trick of buying something I had not been used to buying is what introduced me to jicama, mango, and Greek yogurt. Because of trying Greek yogurt, I have learned to take some frozen strawberries and blueberries and mix them with plain Greek yogurt and a little honey. It is so simple and I have a delicious lunch that seems as delicious as eating pie. I have discovered that jicama is great in a little baggie of raw vegetables and adds variety to what was a boring bag of mini carrots. I still have the carrots but now include jicama, grape tomatoes, green summer squash, red bell pepper slices, and sometimes even yellow tomatoes.

Trying new foods not only helped reduce the frustration at the grocery store but added variety to what I eat. I am less likely to be bored or frustrated with my healthy food choices. I have gotten in touch with my creative side and that, in turn, increases my confidence and self-esteem. It is amazing how all these things are inter-connected. And to top it off, taking home a new food means you get to celebrate the taking of a lovely new MicroStep!

It was extremely hard for me to change my Habit of eating margarine. The truth is that I was eating tons of it without realizing that it was loaded with trans fats. In the beginning, I decided to just switch to butter and not worry about limiting the amounts. MicroSteps, right? Well, that was not so easy because I was used to the taste of the margarine and missed it. Now that I only eat butter, I cannot even imagine what I was thinking. Butter is so much tastier. Our wants do change if given enough time. Eventually, I even decided to reduce my butter intake and continue to work on that each day.

As discussed earlier, when I shared about making my breakfast healthier, reducing butter has been a challenge. My first official MicroStep that focused specifically on reducing butter was to go ahead and put a large pat on my toast but then scrape most if it off after it melted a little. I cannot explain why, but I still feel some mild anxiety at the thought of just putting a dab of butter on my toast. I frequently do the same thing when I'm making scrambled eggs. I put a big glob of butter in the pan and then, after it has melted, I pour most of it out before adding the eggs. Perhaps, someday soon, I will stop wasting butter. Until then, at least, it is not going into my stomach.

Another way I reduce the butter I use with eggs is to eat a hardboiled egg instead of fried eggs or scrambled. In the past, I would put half a stick of butter on a baked potato. After months of MicroSteps, I learned to use parmesan cheese on baked potatoes along with a pat or two of butter, reducing my butter intake. I have also learned to enjoy putting plain Greek yogurt with a little salt on the potato, instead of butter. It tastes like sour cream to me. Sometimes I add a little Balsamic vinegar. It is all about flavor and satisfying our taste buds without creating a panic that causes us to return to negative HRRTs. I am still working on my butter issue.

Learning to cook is work. Increasing your knowledge takes time. Do not expect or try to lose fifty pounds in a couple of months. It will probably happen more quickly than you think but let that be a lovely surprise. Trust your knowledge. Ignore the constantly changing diet fads. It seems like there is always some new warning about what to eat or not eat. Just relax, read what you can about nutrition and food, and then trust yourself. It helps me to stick to fresh non-processed foods.

Are you still struggling with low self-esteem because of your appearance? You do not have to wait until you are at a healthy, average size to begin to change your appearance. You can begin by shopping for clothes that fit your changing size, buying a new pair of shoes, or picking up a piece of jewelry. Scarves, earrings, shoes, watches, a new lipstick color, fit everyone. Just start shopping.

After you lose around 25 pounds and begin to see the benefits of weight loss, it becomes difficult to have the patience to continue to lose weight slowly. At this point, you probably have the willpower to go ahead, jump on a diet fad, and lose weight quickly. My advice is: Do NOT give in!

Losing the Weight for the Last Time

Continue to lose slowly as you work on your HRRTs and self-esteem. The goal is not to lose weight quickly but to lose it for the last time and to live in that healthy, average size body for the rest of your life. This is the turtle's journey. You know, a small turtle may move slowly but it can go many yards in a day if it continues to take those tiny steps.

So change one HRRT at a time and give it a chance to stick solidly before tackling the next HRRT. Rejoice for that new Habit, even if you have not lost weight yet. It is about developing healthy Habits, Routines, Rituals, and Traditions, increasing your knowledge, and trusting the slow process. Imagine that you are building a brick building. You do not pile the bricks all on at once. You lay them carefully and make sure they are bound together with mortar paste before putting the next ones on top. Take this journey the same way, *one brick at a time.*

I started at 315 pounds and when I reached 251 pounds, it was all I could do to continue to take the journey in Micro-Steps. Being close to the 240s was maddening. It was hard to continue to allow the weight to reduce slowly. It would have been so easy to crash diet for a week and lose five to ten pounds quickly. In ten pounds, I knew I would be able to shop in mainstream stores. I wanted so badly to drop the next ten pounds. This is where self-discipline is so critical.

Did you ever think someone would be telling you to lose weight slowly as the key to achieving your goal of permanently reaching a healthy, average size body?

Pick a new HRRT to work on, stick to it, and stay on that track. Do not try to do more than one or two HRRTs at a time. Break them down into MicroSteps and take your time. Create a "to do list" for all those other HRRTs you plan to work on in the future. Lay the list aside and look at it for reassurance from time to time. Add to the list as you become aware of additional negative HRRTs that need change. Trust that you will get to them all in MicroSteps. Resist trying to do everything at once.

Let Them (Not You) Eat Cake

Someday I'll have cake again—just not right now. This became a reassuring thought for me. For a while, it seemed as if cake were everywhere causing me all kinds of conflicts and cravings. Weddings! Birthday Parties! On the Food Network! On the Learning Channel! There were shows about cakes, people talking about cakes, and I just wanted to eat them all and do it all at once.

When you are struggling with cravings, you must ask yourself this question: How often am I craving this and what is the trigger? What is keeping this food, snack, or treat in my head? While there are no foods that are off limits, if you give in to all your cravings and impulses, you will never reach that healthy, average size body. The more awareness you develop regarding your thoughts and actions, the more likely you will be able to identify the trigger and deal with it. Remember, you are a private investigator in your own life. Pay attention to all your thoughts and reactions.

Creating a healthy balanced diet is a challenge after you have been eating in an out of control manner for a long time. How you think about your meals is critical in helping you to establish healthy Habits, Routines, Rituals, and Traditions around food. It is important to remember why you are eating. There is a difference between eating for fuel and eating for pleasure. Eating for fuel needs to be simple, only healthy, quick, and easy. It is about keeping the blood sugar even and the energy level so that you can stay on task and get the job done, whatever is the job.

Eating for pleasure occurs when you are fine dining, celebrating a holiday, or at a special event. It is the time when you spend more money than usual on the meal, when you discuss how delicious is the food, when you enjoy old decadent family recipes, or throw caution to the wind and enjoy the cake at the wedding or other such event.

There is also eating for fuel/pleasure combined. This generally happens at a weekday lunch out, an early dinner out or perhaps a special breakfast at home on the weekend. The fuel/pleasure is about eating for fuel because you know your body needs the nutrition to keep the blood sugar level and your energy up but you are eating in a social setting. The business lunch is a common example. You might order something special from the menu but remember you are primarily eating for fuel and doing it in a social setting. Keep the lid on the impulses; this is not a special event and is not the final meal of your life.

It is important to decide how often you want to eat for pleasure. When you are eating for fuel, it does not need to be the meal magnificent. When I am eating my hardboiled egg and whole grain wheat toast for breakfast, I enjoy it but primarily think of it as fuel. I know that my brain will not do its job with my early morning patients if I have not had some protein and complex carbohydrates. I am trying to get to work on time and not particularly thinking about what I am eating. When I eat out on the weekend at a five star restaurant, I tend to throw caution to the wind and eat almost whatever strikes me in the moment. Since that does not happen daily, I do not worry about it.

When eating for fuel, I may be in a hurry, eating something simple but highly nutritional, and probably less than five hundred calories. Most likely, my focus is on something other than eating, such as work, chores around the house, or perhaps clothes shopping with a friend. Eating for fuel is a daily

Routine that supports a healthy, average size body. Eating for pleasure is an occasional special event with the focus being on the food and perhaps the social engagement or holiday. It is not part of the daily Habits or Routines. I mean, after all, you do not wear your formal attire on daily basis, do you? Why would you eat for pleasure on a daily basis?

When I am eating for fuel/pleasure combined, I try to remember that this is mostly a fuel meal but in a pleasurable setting with good food. If it is a business lunch, I try to stay in the professional mode in my conversation as well as in my food choices and portions sizes. These fuel/pleasure meal situations happen too often for me to throw caution to the wind and use them as an excuse to overeat or make unhealthy food choices. Caution is the word with fuel/pleasure combined meals.

Have you had a bad day? We all have. Some bad days are so bad they would throw even the best of us off track. Others are less severe and just annoy us. Bear in mind, everyone has ups and downs. Not all of them will interfere with your journey to that healthy, average size body. Do not be afraid to check in with a therapist if you cannot get past something that is bothering you.

You are a whole and complex person and unresolved issues are all part of the journey. Deal with what you must, and then ignore the rest. If your imperfections are not affecting your eating, career, social life, family situation, marriage, dating life, or financial choices, then let them go. You can deal with them later if they do start to interfere with your functioning or journey to a healthy, average size body. You don't have to be perfect. None of us is.

You may find that others will not necessarily understand why you take MicroSteps to manage HRRTs. Even after people began to notice that I had lost weight, friends and family continued to try to get me to join a gym, tell me how to diet, and give me weight loss advice. It was not until I had lost over 70 pounds that people finally started *asking me* how to lose weight instead of telling me. It's not easy to ignore everyone around you when you are in a slow lifestyle change. Trust the process. Own your wisdom and you will find a way to deal with the people in your life.

You may not need to address every deeply embedded unresolved issue; however, the daily ups and downs of feelings are another thing. You must not ignore your feelings. If you do, they will create an anxiety that will lead you back to the comfort of the old HRRTs. Whether you go to a therapist or talk to a friend, find a way to process your feelings.

The Celebration List

It was so exciting when I realized I could clap my hands without my chest and stomach being in the way! Pay attention to the changes as they occur and celebrate these even more than the weight loss. Validate the small successes. For example, you had one enchilada and some fruit for lunch instead of three enchiladas with rice. It does not matter that you ate a whole pizza for dinner; you are not working on dinner yet. Celebrate every accomplishment. Nothing is a failure. Just keep putting one foot in front of the other, taking MicroSteps, and you will eventually get to that healthy, average size body. You cannot "fall off the wagon" because no wagon exists.

Pay attention to the changes in your food budget. You will likely notice a reduction. Maybe you can celebrate by spending the savings on new clothes since some of the ones you have may become too large for you. It is so important that you find joy and fun in your life on a daily basis. I know that buying clothes was probably not something you enjoyed in the past when you were greatly overweight, but you will discover that is about to change. Every time I find I need a smaller size, I am all about joy and fun. It is a real good time!

A "celebration list" is literally a list of successes. These successes come from your journey as you are getting to that healthy, average size body. Keep the list somewhere you can look at it easily and quickly but not on the refrigerator. At least for me, I need it out of sight but easily accessible. I do not want it to see it daily. Experiment and do what is best for you.

Here is part of my Celebration List:

- I am not interested in fast food.
- I do not eat in the car anymore.
- I am actually craving fruits and vegetables.
- I am cooking and enjoying cooking.
- I dislike the way my stomach feels when I overeat; therefore, I have stopped overeating.
- I feel much less satisfied when the food I eat is processed, fast food, or unhealthy.
- I crave simple, healthy, well-cooked foods.
- I have more awareness of how my body reacts to what I eat on a meal-by-meal basis.
- My stomach feels empty sometimes and I like that feeling.
- My clothes are hanging on me and I need to go shopping again.

- Less food is filling me up and I cannot eat as much as before.
- I have days and hours when I am so busy with life that I forget to eat. I have to make myself sit down and eat something so that I keep my blood sugar even, never allowing myself to end up so hungry that I return to old HRRTs.

I encourage you to start your own *Celebration List* and keep it where you can see it as often as you need and when you feel as though you need a boost. When I feel the journey to my healthy, average size body is too slow, I read my list and realize that I have already accomplished a mountain of progress. I am moving forward and so are you. The list helps us to remember our progress. It will give you a natural feeling of celebration.

A celebration does not mean that you have to jump up and down and shout. For me, celebration is a quiet, peaceful joy that I feel deeply inside because I know that the *trauma of obesity* is ending in my life and I am now able to move forward without the shame, humiliation, and sadness that goes with feeling so horrible about how you look. Sometimes, I take a breath and smile inside. I have celebrated! No one needs to know that I am rejoicing inside because I declined the dessert at dinner. I know that I am winning the gold medal and it does not matter to me if anyone else sees my celebration, my joy, or my hope. It is there and I am ecstatic!

CHAPTER 8

Productive Exercise

YEARS AGO, I LOVED TO DANCE. Obesity robbed me of that pleasure. I became too large to dance without hurting myself. I have wonderful memories of learning to tap dance, enjoying jazz classes, and taking exercise classes that were mostly dancing. Those were good times. Someday, I may return to dancing; it gives me joy.

I define *productive exercise* as anything that requires physical movement and accomplishes something, including having a good time or increasing your knowledge. Productive exercise could be physical, social, mental, or emotional. The idea is that you are engaging your body, spirit, and mind in an activity that enhances your life.

Physical Exercise

I have never joined a gym and have no plans to do so, unless I decide that it might be fun. Fun is a necessary part of living a healthy balanced life. For me, physical exercise needs to be fun and productive. I get no pleasure out of running on a treadmill that is going nowhere. That's like getting on a cruise ship that never leaves port. Sooner or later, people start to jump off. If I am going to walk or run, then I want to be outside in the fresh air, looking at nature, and enjoying the world around me.

One could argue that walking on a treadmill is productive because it helps you physically. I suppose so, but the fact that the treadmill doesn't go anywhere means I end up quitting. At this point, I may not do a lot of outdoor walking but when I do, I enjoy it fully. My stress goes down and my mind is free to think or ponder. I am not saying you should never go to a gym, if that works for you, but what I am saying is find something that works for you and do it. For me, it needs to be physical movement that I can enjoy while being productive. I am always on the lookout for opportunities to incorporate productive physical exercise into my daily life.

When I weighed 315 pounds, physical movement was a challenge. I remember sitting in my recliner, wanting to get up and do something, but waiting because I knew it would hurt to walk. The physical challenge of getting up and walking discouraged me from moving and doing things. I would tell myself, "Okay, the next commercial you will get up and …" It was depressing. Just standing up from a sitting position was painful and a challenge. At that weight, moving was more about survival and doing what I absolutely had to do rather than the joy of engaging in an activity for fun. Getting to the point where I was willing to do just a little exercise during each commercial was a MicroStep that helped me in the beginning of my journey to a healthy, average size body.

As I began to lose weight, I decided that I wanted to move even more. For a couple of years, I'd been using a motorized cart in the grocery store. I was using it because my knees hurt when I walked. It was embarrassing but I could not make good choices when I was in pain and out of breath. The first physical exercise I did was to *stop using the cart* when I was there for only a couple of items. At first, I was scared that I wouldn't be able to stand in the checkout line without pain. I started on a day that the store had short lines because fewer people were shopping. The first time I tried to shop without the cart, I only bought a loaf of bread. That may not seem like much but it gave me the courage to continue trying. MicroSteps are progress regardless how small. It took a while, but eventually I was able to shop for a whole week's groceries and stand in the checkout line without pain physical pain or exhaustion.

Try to identify MicroSteps that can help you incorporate physical movement into your day. For these to work and become a part of your lifestyle, they must become a part of your automatic and intentional Habits and Routines. Each person has his or her own individual schedule, work environment, daily tasks, and personal idea of what is fun or not fun; therefore, we must each look for our own opportunities for movement. For example, if you sit at a desk in an office for eight hours a day, you might decide to take the long way to the restroom or the break room on a regular basis. Remember, it needs to become something you always do or you will stop doing it at some point and return to Habits and Routines that did not include movement. It needs to be something that you do not dread and that does not feel like you are on an exercise or diet program. It has to be something that you eventually do without thinking because it becomes automatic once incorporated it into your Habits or Routines.

Here are some simple things that help me keep moving:

Herb Garden: I pay a gardener to do the heavy yard work, but I have an herb garden that I like to putter around in myself. It's fun. I am not doing any major gardening but I am bending, cutting, walking and smelling, and enjoying the fresh outside air. Puttering in my herb garden has actually inspired me to do healthier cooking, to get outside more often, to do more walking around in the garden, and to breathe more fresh air. Okay, I know that is not the same as going to the gym with the hard bodies, but it is better than sitting on the sofa watching television.

Housework: I pay a housekeeper to help me with the big stuff; however, there are many chores I do myself and they keep me moving. These tasks include doing my own laundry, keeping the kitchen clean, cleaning the refrigerator, stove, and oven, and running the vacuum a couple times a week. Everything counts, including cleaning out your closet. One day I even did some touch-up painting on the baseboards in my home. That required some bending and using my arms and hands. It may not sound like a lot but I worked up a sweat. I was proud.

Shopping: When I shop for clothes, I spend time walking, looking, and trying things on. I can tell you it feels like a physical workout. In the past, I would wait until I had nothing to wear and then go shopping. I was so out of shape that I could hardly tolerate feeling flushed, the shortness of breath, and the painful knees. Now that I have lost weight, I enjoy my shopping workouts. I also get pleasure from the fact that more clothes fit, my knees don't hurt as much, and my breathing feels normal. When I work up a sweat, I like to think of shopping as my version of going to the gym. Yes, it is productive at the same time. I worked up to this in MicroSteps — but more about that later.

Home and Office: I do pushups to strengthen my upper arms using the island in my kitchen while waiting for something to finish cooking. It is simple. Step two feet away from the counter, lean forward, put your hands on the counter, and do pushups. It takes very little time and amazingly enough my arms are getting stronger and I can see a little muscle starting to develop.

Another simple MicroStep I took when going to work was simply to carry my purse, laptop, and lunch in my hands instead of putting them in a carrier cart and rolling them the easy way. I loved that no one knew I was exercising. This worked for several months but eventually I had to return to the cart because of arthritis in my lower back. You see, you need to experiment, see what works for you, and build your own Habits and Routines that you can incorporate into a permanent lifestyle, without hurting yourself or doing something you hate and thus consequently quit.

Adding productive physical exercise to your daily life has benefits other than just weight management. You may notice that you are getting more of your chores done and having more time for a social life. After all, if you have been getting up during every commercial while watching your favorite television show, then you may have cleaned the kitchen, run the vacuum, folded the laundry, made the beds, or even repaired that screen door that has been calling you.

You can divide your grocery shopping into two trips and that will give you even more opportunity for productive walking. How about washing your own car and letting the kids help? Are you getting the idea? This is all about making your life easier by using productive physical exercise to help you manage your physical health, all the while reducing the stress of having all those chores waiting for you.

Poppy, my beautiful long-haired white and orange female cat, helped my exercise routine by deciding she disliked the litter box even the slightest bit dirty. She began to do her business outside the litter box on a mat. This caused me to have to bend more, do more laundering of the mats, and to have to walk to the bathroom more often to clean the box. Instead of looking at it as an annoyance, I decided to make lemonade out of lemons and think of it as a new productive exercise. Every movement counts. I just think

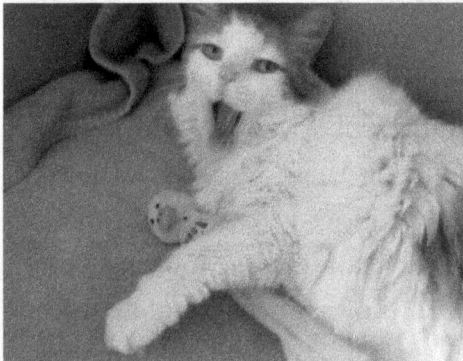

Poppy, "Hey mom, the litter box is dirty! Think I'll use the mat."

of Poppy as my little furry trainer. The cleaner I keep the box, the more she does her business in the box.

Then there is my other cat, Oliver, a large handsome shorthaired male with white and orange fur. He weighs about seventeen pounds and loves it when I stretch him out, lift him high into the air the way they do at cat shows, and then do a few bench presses. He is too heavy to do many lifts but I do a couple at a time. Poppy and Oliver are my trainers. Poppy keeps me walking and bending; Oliver builds my muscles. Way to go furry training team!

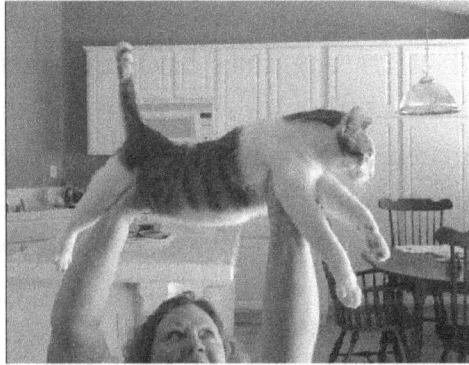

Oliver, "Nice view, mom—a little higher, please."

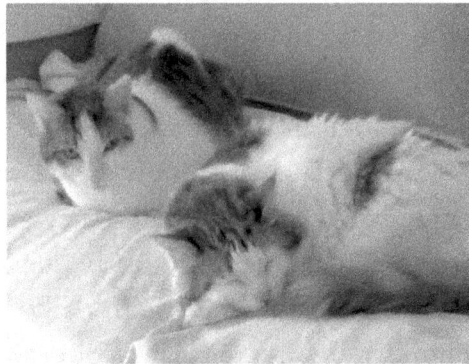

Oliver and Poppy: My personal trainers are ready for naps.

One night on the way home from work, I decided that I wanted to do a little walking. It had been a long day at work and it seemed as though I had been sitting forever. The day was hot and I had no interest in sweating so I stopped at the nearest store and figured I would walk and shop. After all, shopping is one of my favorite exercises.

Dick's Sporting Goods store was the nearest so I parked, went in, and began my walk. I enjoyed looking at all the things I will never use such as fishing and golf equipment. Then I saw the barbells, weights, and dumbbells (an exercise weight in the form of a metal bar with a metal disk or ball at each end). I tried lifting some of them and discovered that I could safely manage five pounds in each hand. Being out of shape and having arthritis can be limiting. I purchased two for home and two for the office. They were around six dollars each and that is far less than a gym membership.

My work as a therapist and writer requires hours of sitting, talking, and typing. I now enjoy stretching and doing a five-minute workout with the dumbbells several times a day. It is quick, easy, and helps me build strength. It also seems to help with stress management because I am not sitting hour after hour without taking a movement break.

You might be asking, "How are the dumbbells productive?" I don't know. I just know that I saw them, got this idea, and enjoy using them. Perhaps they are productive because of the stress management factor. It doesn't matter. I am having fun with them and using them daily. I can do them while on the phone, watching television, or even standing outside looking at my herb garden.

Dumbbells were easy to add to my daily Routine. They are a MicroStep in beginning physical exercise and they help me build up my muscles. The sales clerk at the store tried to get me to buy ten-pound weights. He said the five pounds were too easy. I knew that I would never use the ten pounds because they hurt my hands and shoulders after just a few lifts. I chose to start with five pounds, MicroSteps, because I knew that would lead to success and be a permanent change in my Routine. It has been exciting to experience the increased strength in my arms.

When you are very obese and just starting to integrate productive physical exercise into your day, even small efforts may seem like a challenge due to the pain and effort required just to move. This is a perfect opportunity to take it in MicroSteps. Perhaps, you can vacuum one extra time a week to improve the look of your house. Maybe you can walk outside to pick up the newspaper instead of asking your spouse or one of your kids to get it for you. Do what you can and be proud of each small thing you do, build on that, and continue to do one MicroStep at a time until each becomes a Habit or Routine. Before you know it, you will have added a whole collection of productive exercises to your lifestyle. Yes, it is all about the MicroSteps.

Look at your physical Habits, Routines, Rituals, and Traditions. Determine where you might make a change that would add some intentional productive physical exercise into your life. Choose the smallest possible MicroStep at first and start there. For me, that first MicroStep was doing those pushups against the island in my kitchen. Stop comparing yourself to the thin person who tells you the answer is to join a gym or take a long walk. That's fine for them; but for you, doing five to ten pushups at the kitchen counter is just as important. My small MicroSteps of productive physical exercise are a way for me to get my body moving and to do it without advertising that I am exercising.

Social Exercise

Social Exercise is productive and critical in maintaining a healthy balanced life. This means you need to talk to people. Get in the car and go somewhere. It does not matter what you do, as long as you have a Habit, Routine, Ritual, or Tradition that includes social interactions with others. If you have been isolating, then you will probably need to begin in MicroSteps. Perhaps your first MicroStep is going to a Starbucks and speaking to the person preparing your coffee. You might decide to walk to the end of your street for a brief conversation with a neighbor. Perhaps you pause to speak to another parent when you pick your child up from school. MicroSteps can lead you into new productive social exercise without causing the anxiety or panic that stems from low self-esteem about how you look and what you perceive others may think of you.

If you have been a social butterfly, then you may need to evaluate your social activities and relationships to determine if they are supporting healthy HRRTs. You may need to decide whether your social life is interfering with a healthy lifestyle. Do you eat badly when you are alone or when you're with others? Are you a closet eater or a public eater?

My own overeating occurred both when I was alone and with other people who were overeaters. When I was living in Los Angeles, my eating was healthier because the people I associated with were fairly health conscious. When I moved to Bakersfield, California, my eating became less healthy because I was around people who enjoyed more fattening foods, such as sodas with sugar and sweets. I had fewer friends in Bakersfield. There were fewer opportunities to go places where I needed to dress nicely, such as fine dining. The more casual environment meant I could dress in oversized cheap clothes and still go out to eat in Bakersfield. This was generally at fast food places or restaurants that were not much healthier than fast food. My Habits and Routines changed in a negative way. My social exercises were not supporting a healthy, average size body. I began to pile on the pounds. Ask yourself the following questions:

- Are you going out to eat with other large-size people who like to "eat large" with you?
- Are you going to restaurants that do not offer healthy choices?
- Do your social and family times revolve around heavy fattening meals and drinking alcohol?
- Do others pressure you when you try to eat healthy or decline alcohol?
- Are there cakes, candies, pies, fried foods, chips and dips at every family event?
- Are your social outings so rare that when you do go out you order everything in sight?
- Can you go to a movie without an enormous serving of fattening theater popcorn and an extra large soda?
- Do your social outings involved physical movement?

Busy at the Barbeque

Not long ago I had a barbeque at my house with twenty guests and tons of food, all cooked by a fabulous chef. I was so busy and worked so hard physically to attend to the preparations and guests that I rarely had a chance to sit down. I felt as though I'd had a physical workout. I skipped lunch and didn't get around to enjoying any of the barbeque food until later in the afternoon. Yes, I ate a little of most of the dishes, including pie for dessert, but I ended up eating less than my normal day's intake of calories. I love it when productive social and physical exercises combine to create a magnificent day!

Mental Exercise

You will only get out of your mind that which you put into your mind. If all you do is sit around and read romance novels, you will not learn algebra. A romance novel now and then is okay, but your mind needs a healthy balance of information input on a daily basis. You get out what you put in.

Productive mental exercise is a critical part of developing a healthy lifestyle. In this process of taking back your power by creating a permanent lifestyle change that supports a healthy, average size body, you cannot leave your intellect out of the process. Knowledge is power. You are in the battle of your life, fighting for your life, and you need the power of the kind of knowledge that will support your ultimate goal. Find a class on nutrition, a book with exciting recipes, or learn to research on your computer. Get in the game!

You might need to begin in MicroSteps to get you started. If you are addicted to television and watch it many hours a day, your first MicroStep might be watching a half-hour cooking show on *The Food Network*. It's still television; however, it is increasing your knowledge at the same time. Perhaps the next step is to watch a healthy cooking show twice a week or even once a day. It may inspire you to try a new dish. Cooking a new, healthy dish is a lovely way to create a new healthy Habit or Routine. The chef on the cooking show might talk about a utensil that you don't own. Since mental exercise needs to include some physical movement at least part of the time, consider this possibility. You decide you need to get out of the house for some productive physical exercise (shopping) in order to purchase the new utensil. While at the store buying the new utensil, you remember that the TV chef discussed a cookbook. You decide to go to the bookstore to buy the cookbook. While at the bookstore, you see a book on nutrition. It is on a high shelf, so you use a stepstool to help you reach the book. You buy the nutrition book. All of a sudden you are productively walking, shopping, and increasing your knowledge. Now, you've got it!

If you don't watch the cooking shows, buy the books, bring them home, or read them, you won't learn what they have to teach you, so there's no chance of getting the help they offer. If you don't buy vegetables and bring them home, you won't eat them; this is the same idea. Start with one book. Buy it. Bring it home. Lay it on a table. Say to yourself that you have taken a MicroStep and know that others will follow. Celebrate that you have taken that one MicroStep. You bought the book. Once you start to input knowledge, it will become addictive. I promise.

Productive mental exercise is not only about cooking or nutrition. It is about learning anything that stimulates you mentally and gets you involved in life. Perhaps you are having problems in your marriage or with friends. Learning more about interpersonal relationships and working through things with a psychotherapist can be productive mental exercise; it can also be emotional exercise. Perhaps you are interested in computers, finishing your college degree, or taking an art class—all are opportunities for productive mental exercise. Some include getting in the car and going somewhere to accomplish that mental exercise. Go for it. Become an active participant in your life.

Emotional Exercise

Productive emotional exercise is critical if you want to become a healthy, average size person. Emotional exercise is productive when you are participating in an activity or relationship that positively touches your heart, your soul, or your emotions. You could do this via volunteer work at a senior citizen facility, having sex with your lover, or teaching a class at your church or temple. You might consider coaching your child's team, being the Cub Scout Leader, getting back into the dating game, or doing some personal shopping for someone who is ill. It is productive on so many levels because you are off the sofa, physically exercising, involved with another person, experiencing empathy, feeling frustration, having a moment of joy, feeling useful, and in the mainstream of life.

Begin as slowly, in MicroSteps, as you need to, but look for ways to get your emotions involved in your life. Are you afraid of feelings and afraid to share them? This might be something to discuss with a psychotherapist, or maybe you just need to start slowly. Be not afraid; the only emotions that will hurt you are the ones you stuff. Stuffing emotions inside will lead to unhealthy behaviors that often include stuffing yourself with food. It is important to get emotions to work for you instead of against you, if you are going to achieve that healthy, average size body.

You may need to use productive physical exercise to help you manage an emotion that is giving you a difficult time.

Gardening, walking the dog, or mowing the lawn can help you deal with anger or anxiety. Slug a pillow or a punching bag to siphon off some of your frustration. Combining productive physical, social, mental, and emotional exercises is unavoidable and part of creating a healthy balanced lifestyle.

Emotional exercise is challenging. While you need to move physically to get out and do whatever you have chosen to do, you are also investing your heart, feelings, and spirit in the experience. It can feel like a major risk; however, it has the possibility of being life changing. Now *that* is productivity!

Start with something that feels easy and non-threatening. Remember my alcoholic patient who spent weeks just driving by the Alcoholics Anonymous (AA) meeting site because he was too afraid to walk into a meeting? This brave soul ended up speaking at many of the meetings and even becoming the Secretary of one of them. In the beginning, bravery may mean simply waving to a neighbor. That may be only a MicroStep but it is a big step in the right direction.

Just Do Something

Start somewhere. Do something. Anything you do will take you to the next step. Be proud of whatever you do that helps you move forward. It is not a contest. There is no teacher grading you. No one will know how hard you have to work to take that first MicroStep. It can be your secret and someday when you are an average, healthy size person, you can tell them how you did it.

A healthy life is a dance and must include getting up, getting out, getting informed, and getting involved. If you want to maintain healthy Habits, Routines, Rituals, and Traditions that support a healthy, average size body, you must get up off the sofa, get out of the house, add to your knowledge, and get involved with other people. The rest will happen all in good time. Remember, everything counts. It is all about productive exercise in MicroSteps.

There is a bowling alley out there with your name on it. There is a dance studio with room for one more student in their jazz class. Ask a friend or significant other to take you to a Ballroom Dance Class. Catch a movie. Go for a bike ride. It does not matter what you do, as long as you do something. Become a dancer in the mainstream of life!

CHAPTER 9

It Is Not a Plateau!

TRASH THE SCALES; I WANT OFF! After losing sixty-four pounds, I suddenly stopped and could not seem to lose an ounce more. After about four months of this, I became deeply discouraged. I did not understand why this was happening. I began to wonder if perhaps that old myth about *hitting a plateau* was true after all. I'd always debunked that idea. Now, thinking that I had hit a plateau after all made me feel powerless. Had I reached the end of the slow-but-steady weight loss that I'd been experiencing each month for the past few years? Since *slow-but-steady* is the whole point of this book, I was upset at the idea that there might be a glitch in it! I was even more upset that I might never reach my healthy, average size body.

Then it got even worse. I would get on the scale only to find that I had gained two or three pounds. The next day I would find I had lost two to five pounds. I was scared. I thought I was eating well, nothing had changed, but my weight was all over the place. When I looked in the mirror, I could see weight loss and my clothes were getting too big again. What was going on? I could not figure it out.

Disheartened, I slowly began to snack a little at night and then I blamed the erratic weight on the snacking. The snacks were fruit and yogurt but nonetheless I blamed the snacking.

One day I got on the scale and saw a five-pound increase. I simply could not believe it. I got back on the scale again. This time it said I had lost three pounds! I weighed again and came up with a different number. Finally, I realized that the scale was broken. It had taken me over three months to question my scale and realize it was wrong. Relieved, I purchased a professional doctor's scale (the kind with the weights that move) and now I have an accurate weight each day.

I had spent all these months questioning myself and feeling as though I was failing. Once I began to weigh on an accurate scale, I also discovered I had actually only lost sixty pounds. That was fine; at least I knew where I was and how to move forward. The scale was now consistent. Because of the inaccurate scale, I had been eating wrong amounts but thinking I was eating okay. I had not been able to identify HRRTs that needed my attention. Lesson learned.

In addition to the broken scale at home, I had been weighing at work but at different times, on different scales, wearing different clothes (different weights), and after eating or drinking a lot of water. This was also creating confusion. In the beginning of my journey, my home scale had been new and accurate; it was also a cheap scale. Initially, I weighed on the doctor's scale at work and at the same time each day. I had gotten careless with the weighing process, as my confidence increased. That was a mistake. As you can see, knowing your accurate weight is critical in helping you learn to adjust what you are eating and figure out what HRRTs need your attention. After having the new scale for a week, reevaluating what I had been eating, and making some easy adjustments, I set out to discover what had caused me to stop losing weight in the first place.

There is No Plateau

After solving the weight tracking mystery, I decided to go back to the beginning and examine what I was eating. I felt resistant to taking another MicroStep toward change; however, it had to be a Habit or Routine preventing my progress to that healthy, average size body. I had gotten overly confident because the new HRRTs had become easy and I had not realized that I would need to make additional changes to continue to lose. Two things had caused me to be stuck: The broken scale and my eating both needed changing.

In trying to figure out what was happening, I found a couple of problems. I had allowed the calories to increase. Remember, you need to monitor the calories every so often, even though you are not counting them daily. Calories are a reality in weight management.

The healthy brand of tortilla chips I had been buying had increased from a handful every couple of weeks to daily. Additionally, I had started buying packages of shredded cheeses and was using large handfuls on salads, pastas, meats, in my healthy chili, and even in some soups. I had had some passing thoughts about this but did not want to admit, even to myself, that I had created some negative HRRTs with cheese and tortilla chips. Tortilla chips with melted cheese had become a negative Habit that had slipped into my daily Routine, as well as adding cheese to other foods. These negative HRRTs added up to enough additional calories to stop the weight loss and prevent me from moving toward that healthy, average size body.

I decided to take MicroSteps to address these new negative Habits. I had not realized that new negative Habits or Routines could sneak into my new healthy eating HRRTs. The first MicroStep I took was to buy a smaller bag of tortilla chips and to allow myself to eat them only every other day. Eventually, I was able to stop buying the tortilla chips altogether. The second MicroStep was more difficult. I love cheese, especially melted cheese. I decided that I would be eating less cheese if I only bought the blocks of cheese and shredded it myself. That worked. I do not have the patience to shred a large handful. I tend to shred an ounce or two and toss it onto whatever I am eating. Problem solved for now; however, I realized at this point that I would need to continue to monitor my HRRTs and do the random spot check on calories as we discussed earlier.

Here is the lesson: You must continue to monitor and change your HRRTs until you actually reach that healthy, average size body. You see, *there is no plateau.* You simply stop losing when what you are eating is supporting your current weight. That means you must take in less food or fewer calories to continue to lose. The cheese and tortillas were adding too many calories to my diet and that caused me to stop losing. Because I believed my eating had become healthy and I had not looked at the details of my food intake for a couple of months, I had not realized that new negative Habits had snuck into my daily Routine. Believing that I had hit a plateau caused me to slip into denial about what I was eating; it also caused me to trust a broken scale.

Self-Perception Confusion

Looking back, after I'd lost forty-four pounds, I felt thin even though I still weighed 271 pounds. I could feel my hipbones and ribs. I'd been watching *What Not to Wear* on TV, figured I'd learned a thing or two about how to dress fashionably, and had even bought some new clothes. One morning, dressed in new clothes, I was excited as I headed off to the office, thinking I looked stylish and even a little chic.

While waiting for the elevator at the clinic where I work, I caught a glimpse of my reflection in the highly polished metal doors. I realized, with great disappointment, that I did not look as good as I thought. When I'd looked in the mirror at home, it had not connected in my brain as it did at that moment in the reflection in the elevator door. I had to face the fact that I was still very obese. I guess I knew it all along; I know my weight, my size, and my measurements. I also knew that over-coming the discouragement that clouded my brain after that quick glimpse of my reflection was not going to be easy. I had to force myself to put my thoughts aside, go in, and meet with my first patient.

This was to be one of many times that I experienced such a disconnect between feeling thin, while still having almost a hundred pounds left to lose to get to an average size.

It happened again after I had lost fifty-two pounds. Not only had I been feeling thin, but I had also been experiencing an incredible increase in my physical energy. My clothes were hanging on me; it was time to go shopping again. I was even concerned that a beautiful velvet jacket I had purchased months earlier, at an upscale store, was going to be too big before the weather turned cool enough to wear it. When I arrived at work one day, a psychiatrist colleague showed me a picture that she had taken of me at a recent event. I was surprised and discouraged to see that I still looked very obese. Again, there was that mental disconnect between my intellectual understanding of how much more weight I needed to lose and how great I was feeling.

It is often difficult to continue with this slow journey of MicroSteps, while you are allowing your body to adjust to the fact that it is only getting enough fuel to maintain an average healthy size. When you are only losing one to three pounds a month, it can feel as though you are getting nowhere.

I share this with you to prepare you for possible feelings of frustration. I want you to understand that this is to be expected. It takes time for self-awareness to catch up with your body and the continuing changes. Perhaps you have lost a lot of weight but you still feel fat instead of thin. Perhaps you look in the mirror and see large when the tape measure says otherwise. We are all different but we share one thing: As we lose large amounts of weight, we may experience confusion in our self-perception that will take time to resolve.

Years ago, when I was beginning to gain large amounts of weight, I was always bumping into things. Walking between chairs in a restaurant was a challenge. I would see a space and think I could walk through it easily but then my larger size body would bump into the chairs. I had bruises on my hips for months, until my brain finally connected to the actual size of my body. Lately, I have noticed that I can walk between chairs more easily and that some chairs are a much better fit when I sit down in them.

Healthy Celebrations

There is no question, it is exciting to begin to lose weight and to feel better physically after being so large for so long. It is natural to want to acknowledge the success and I want you to celebrate each MicroStep. For many people, celebrations include food. What do we do when someone has a birthday, a graduation, a baby shower, a wedding? We have cake! We toast with champagne! We think, "Now that I have lost some pounds, I will stop tonight and pick up a pizza; after all, I have earned it." Whoa! Consider this: You have earned much more than an eating binge or a cake; you have earned the right to live happier in a healthy, average size body.

This is where the Habits, Routines, Rituals, and Traditions come into play again. It is critical to discover ways to be proud, celebrate success, and feel the joy of becoming a healthy person again without using sweets, pizza, fast food, or even going to a five star restaurant as a means of celebration. That is not the message you want to give your subconscious. It is better to eat these foods at a time when there is no emotion or celebration connected with them. It will take some of their power away.

Your new Habits, Routines, Rituals, and Traditions are very young at this stage and need protection. As you are on this journey, you must continue to look for unhealthy HRRTs that sabotage your ability to maintain a healthy body. It is also important to identify behaviors that are creating new unhealthy HRRTs that could become problems in the future. For example, my friend likes a certain type of soda, so I started buying some to keep on hand for her—until I caught myself drinking one, then two, and suddenly I realized I was developing a new Habit! I stopped right away and kept extra bottled waters on hand instead.

Once you identify negative Habits, Routines, Rituals, and Traditions, be they old ones or new ones, begin slowly in MicroSteps to replace them with the healthy HRRTs that support your new healthier lifestyle.

The Need for Comfort

We all have stress in our lives and find those moments when we just need to be comforted. We may find that comfort in a good book, our favorite television show, or a box of chocolates. We all need to find something to provide that comfort but it is important that we make it as healthy as possible.

After the pre-operation appointments for a minor surgery, I felt scared, stressed, and anxious. I decided to have some good ole comfort food. That night, I had pizza for dinner, ate a couple of slices, and felt no interest in the rest. The next day, I had fried chicken with macaroni and cheese but threw most of it away because it made my stomach hurt. It just didn't meet the need I felt for comfort. The next meal, I tried salad with tortilla soup and realized to my surprise that they had become my new comfort foods. At last, I felt the calm that in the past unhealthy comfort foods would have provided. Later, I had one scoop of Haagen-Dazs ice cream and found it to be nice and comforting. One scoop was all I wanted and it was delicious. This slip helped me realize that I had changed from the inside out, literally. To my amazement, I found that what was once a comfort food for me was no longer comforting. My needs and wants had changed.

A colleague of mine wrote a book titled *Count it as a Vegetable and Move On!* (See the Resource Section.) My favorite part of this book is the title and I've often used it as a kind of mantra to say to myself whenever I eat something that, in the past, would have filled me with guilt. I simply say aloud, *"Just count it as a vegetable and move on!"* I then congratulate myself for how well I'm doing. It helps keep up my spirits. It works like magic in helping me avoid beating myself up when I am less than perfect on my journey toward my goal of a healthy, average size body.

It is important to remember that we find comfort in the familiar and in Routines. The reason that fried chicken and macaroni with cheese used to comfort me is because they made up my primary diet for many years. They were my Habit, a family Routine, and a Southern Tradition. The tortilla soup is a new comfort food because it has become my new Habit. Again, there is so much power in Habits, Routines, Rituals, and Traditions. What a trip!

Behaving *"As If"*

The song lyrics, *"Whistle a happy tune, make believe you're brave,"* came to my mind as a way to deal with the emotional ups and downs of this phase of the journey towards a healthy, average size body. I decided to behave *as if* I were beautiful and well dressed. I decided to believe that if I lived and acted like an average size, well-dressed person, I would eventually become such. I was determined to continue my journey without allowing its slowness to cause a derailment.

How was I able to make such a decision? It helped that I had been keeping an Excel spreadsheet of my weight for over a year. This allowed me to see my progress visually and to understand that I am moving forward. I also reminded myself that my body may not look average size today but I am feeling and moving better than I have for years. That helped.

This is a time to use those self-observation skills. Take some time to remember all the changes you have made, remember how it was before you took your first MicroStep, and think about the Habits, Routines, Rituals, and Traditions you have changed. Whether you have lost two pounds, twenty pounds, or two hundred pounds, the journey is the same. You must simply continue to put one foot in front of the other and walk the path slowly. Do not panic if you are not losing weight quickly, or even at all for a while, simply continue becoming more aware of the negative HRRTs that are causing you to be overweight and take MicroSteps to change them.

This is also a good time to use some of your check-up tools. Do you need to get out the tape measure? Should you do a calorie check, just to make sure you are not fooling yourself about how much you are eating? Is it time to go shopping and buy a new outfit to celebrate the weight you have lost, or just to celebrate your intentions to get to that healthy, average size body? Perhaps you need to review Chapter 6 to remind yourself how to confirm your progress. Have you identified a specific tiny MicroStep on which you are working today?

Just to let you know: I wrote this chapter while I was feeling discouraged and frustrated with the slowness of my journey to becoming an average size. It seemed as though my insides were sophisticated and stylish but would never match the outside that was still obese and dressed in cheap supersized clothes. The reason I continued to write the chapter while discouraged was so that you would know you are not alone. As long as you do not give up, you will find your way to being an average size. With traditional diets, people lose quickly and then regain the weight. You are on a different road.

The journey of the HRRTs is not only slow but requires continual evaluation and adjustment. That is radically different from a traditional diet where someone tells you how to eat and when to eat. This is your journey and you are in charge of making it work. That can be scary and frustrating, almost like finding your way in the dark. Just don't give up. As long as you are taking MicroSteps, you will get there; once arrived, you will have that healthy, average size body forever.

Mental and Emotional Toughness

As you've discovered by now, this is not an easy journey. It is not for the emotionally weak, the feeble of spirit, the impatient, or for the person who gives up easily. Regardless, you can still succeed. How do you build up mental and emotional toughness? Actually, they work together. One way is to get up, get out, and do something that requires movement. The worst thing you can do is sit at home, watch television, and think about what you would like to do if only you were thin. This is a time to dance! You may need to review Chapter 8 to get some ideas for activities. You do not need to be thin in order to participate in social activities, learn something new, or physically move. One way out of discouragement is to choose an activity or behavior that you believe will help you move forward and begin in MicroSteps. Focus on making today a good day instead of worrying about what will happen in the future. The Twelve-Step Programs have it right. If you are struggling, take it one day at a time or even five minutes at a time.

You may have times when you stop losing weight; however, remember that you need to stop and check what you are eating, look at the negative HRRTs that may be preventing your success, and make the adjustments in MicroSteps. These slow weight loss times can cause doubts and be discouraging. Make sure you have an accurate scale and be honest with yourself about what you are eating and doing.

You do not need to be without doubts. We all have moments of doubt. You can keep going in spite of them, and in spite of your fear that you will never reach your healthy, average size body. Many believe, *"…if you have faith the size of a mustard seed…nothing will be impossible to you."* (New American Standard Bible, Matthew 17:20). Do you know how small a mustard seed is? It is very tiny! All you need is to believe just enough to continue to make MicroSteps to healthier Habits, Routines, Rituals, and Traditions. You may actually be surprised as you lose weight and see for yourself that this slow journey of the HRRTs actually works.

CHAPTER 10

Grooming and Public Presentation

SITTING IN A BUSINESS MEETING years ago, I remember looking down at my enormous body covered in baggy super-size clothing and thinking that I wanted to keep my mouth shut rather than draw attention to myself. Unfortunately, I was running the meeting and did not have that option. Feeling humiliated by my appearance robbed me of the courage I needed to address the challenging issues in the meeting.

How you groom and dress for work, home, social situations, and all other events has a significant impact on how that day goes. Grooming and style play a major role in determining which people seek you out and how they perceive you. The way you present your physical self may either destroy self-esteem or give it a big boost. These days, it takes courage and confidence to make it professionally. Your public presentation can either make or break your career. Men and women both struggle with this reality.

The way you dress influences every aspect of your life. This includes how the teachers react to you in high school, how the professors in college see you, the quality of reference letters that will be written to help you get that first job, how you are perceived in a job interview, and even the way you approach a job interview. People who are not properly dressed for a job interview are likely to be more anxious and this may lose them the job as a result. What you wear, and how you groom yourself, can determine with whom you hang out, the social activities in which you choose to participate, and what type of people you date or even marry.

This chapter is going to address grooming, how you take care of your personal hygiene, and what you can do to look your best even before you have lost one pound. Grooming is an area where people slack off when they get discouraged and people who are overweight or obese are often discouraged. Everything is difficult when you hate the size of your body—especially grooming and style.

Daily Grooming

It is almost impossible not end up in a depression when you are extremely large. Depression is common among the obese. Being overweight causes a reduction in energy and motivation. People often find themselves sitting on the sofa, watching television, not taking a daily shower, wearing nightclothes all day, isolating socially, not changing clothes for days, and becoming even more discouraged. It's a vicious circle. When you live your life this way, you end up feeling hopeless. Your self-esteem is at the bottom of a pit so deep you do not even see the sunshine above. It is a horrible place to be and to live. There is a way out but you must start somewhere. I hope that by now you have been working on your HRRTs and MicroSteps toward positive change. If not, it is never too late to *get up* and change your life.

Yep, I said, "*Get up.*" You cannot move forward sitting on the sofa and feeling like a failure. Below are four tasks you will need to accomplish on a daily basis to help you begin to feel better about yourself and your life. You need to do these daily, even if you are not leaving the house.

1. Take a shower, shave (legs or face), and brush your teeth.
2. Wash your hair at least every other day.
3. Get out of your nightclothes put on clean day clothes.
4. Comb and style your hair.

I know it is not easy when you have totally given up. For people who get up and get dressed every day, these four steps may seem ridiculously simple. For people who have given up on ever reaching a healthy, average size body, I might as well have asked you to climb a mountain. You may need to take Micro-Steps to be able to accomplish these four daily tasks. As long as you start, you are making progress. Take a MicroStep and then celebrate your success—but not with food. Perhaps one morning you decide to wash your face. Call that the first MicroStep. Remember, the HRRTs will change in MicroSteps and each MicroStep is a move forward.

Let's say you have been getting up, taking a shower, and getting dressed every day. There are still questions: What are you putting on? Are you dressing your best with what you have? I understand that when you are feeling unhappy with your size it's difficult to go ahead and make the best of what you do have. However, little things you can do to begin to present yourself in your best light will make a world of difference in how you feel throughout the day. When you feel good about what you are wearing and are enjoying a cleanly shaven face or fresh make-up, you will eat healthier—if for no other reason than you need less comfort food.

Okay, I know most of you men are not wearing makeup. Nonetheless, it is time to use a little moisturizer on your face and some after-shave or cologne. Do it daily, even if you are not leaving the house. Your face will thank you and it will lift your spirits. Many grooming items will work whether you are a large, small, or an average size. After-shave or cologne could be that first MicroStep to a healthy, average size body.

Women, go ahead and put on the make-up. Frankly, I consider putting on make-up as important as brushing my teeth. Even if you are just going to the grocery store or to the cleaners, putting on make-up will help you feel better about how you look. I know it is hard to shop for clothing when it seems like nothing fits but make-up can be used regardless of your physical size. You will be surprised at how much a little makeup will do for your confidence. If you are not going out, at least clean your face daily and apply moisturizer.

If you are not sure about how to apply make-up, get someone at the make-up counter at a department store to help you. Most of the sales clerks are glad to give free lessons because they want you to buy their products. Take advantage of the opportunity to increase your knowledge. Remember, knowledge is power and the more you know the more confidence you will have. The more confidence you have, the less bumpy the path to your healthy, average size body.

Next, adding accessories such as a scarf or jewelry is another opportunity to feel better quickly. There are caps, hats, scarves, interesting watches, rings, and interesting shoes available to both men and women. You do not need to overdo it. Just a little glitter or gold, or a scarf of fine wool or silk makes a statement. The jewelry may be "costume," the "cashmere" scarf may just be a "look-alike," and the shoes may not be a name brand, but they may help you feel better about your appearance.

Start to dress your best before you've even lost that first pound. Act *as if* you care about yourself. The irony is that the sooner you begin to dress *as if* you care about yourself, the more you will actually care, and the better you will feel. The better you feel, the better you will eat. Your confidence will begin to increase and you are on your way to healthier HRRTs and a healthy, average size body.

Men, even you "manly men" out there who may scoff at this kind of focus on grooming—please realize that men who are well groomed and develop their own dressing style move forward in dating, marriages, careers, and all aspects of their lives. Get a facial or talk to the person who cuts your hair about those nose and ear hairs that you've been ignoring. You may want to have a professional shave. And don't even get me started on how much a professional massage can do for your mood. You will also want to take it in MicroSteps. Perhaps the first step is to get on the internet and find out more about male grooming tips. It is a MicroStep and less threatening than walking into a salon for a grooming lesson.

Women, as you're going through your day, check your hair or make-up. The afternoon people in your life need to see you at your best as well as the morning folks. People who care about how they look check themselves when they go to the restroom or after they eat lunch. You will not make a very good impression in a meeting with spinach in your teeth. Beginning to touch up during the day so that you always look your best will help you move forward. How can you begin to live *as if*, when you are looking sloppy?

A few years ago, I attended an evening wine and cheese party given by the head of a school district. There were many officials from the district present, as well as other professionals from the community. It was a lovely house with a fabulous backyard. While I was still at my largest, about 315 pounds, I had dressed to the best of my ability. I felt good at the event. I enjoyed sitting around the fireplace in the backyard talking with colleagues. The host offered the opportunity to make S'mores, a traditional campfire treat consisting of a roasted marshmallow and a layer of chocolate sandwiched between two pieces of graham cracker. I accepted, and we all enjoyed the childhood treats, while sitting by the fireplace. It was fun!

Later, on the way home, I looked down and saw graham cracker crumbs all over the top of my black sweater. I was mortified. In addition to being the largest person in the room, I had crumbs on my sweater. Why hadn't someone told me? Why hadn't I looked down to brush them off before going back into the house? Other people had participated in the S'mores but I hadn't seen crumbs on their sweaters. Had I been so lost in the sweet treat that I had forgotten to take care of my appearance? It remains one of my most embarrassing moments.

You may not choose to wear make-up but there are plenty of other grooming tasks. Keep those finger nails clean and shaped nicely, brush your hair, check or brush your teeth after lunch, and do something about that unwanted nose hair. Men, you may even want to grab a quick shave before an important meeting. In other words, keep your face, hair, and your hands presentable. Keep your clothes clean and fresh. You will be surprised how much better you will feel and how your confidence will increase. Self-confidence is a powerful tool in moving forward to that healthy, average size body.

Impact of Obesity on Job Interviews and Promotions

I have been the obese person interviewing for a job; I have been the employer interviewing an obese person. Either side of the desk is uncomfortable. When I was the obese person interviewing for a job, my low self-image caused me to be more nervous and less confident in my ability to interview. When I was interviewing the obese person for a job, I could not help but wonder what was not working in his or her life. In some cases, I was more obese than the large person I was interviewing. Yet, I still found myself biased. It seemed that the obese people I interviewed were nervous and thus unable to come across as professional as did the average size interviewee. While I am sure others have had different experiences, this was my experience.

I admit this was a bias on my part. I felt horrible and saw myself as a hypocrite. There I was trying to convince my potential boss that I was qualified for the job regardless of my size, and yet I could not give a potential employee the same open-mindedness. I think that is because being obese had destroyed my own self-image and confidence to the point that I did not believe my own spin about being equal regardless of size.

Job interviewing is a challenge no matter what your weight. Being uncomfortable in your own skin may come across to the potential employer or cause you to struggle in the interview. Even if the potential employer is completely unbiased, you are likely still hard on yourself. That may cause you to struggle in the interview.

It is, however, not a hopeless task. There are things you can do to help yourself before you reach that healthy, average size body. Make sure you have prepared for the interview in terms of knowing the company and the job you are seeking. Be on time but not too early. Prepare for the questions you will likely need to answer and have all your paperwork in perfect order. Those things will impress regardless of size. Most importantly, make sure you are dressed for the job for which you are interviewing. It may take some work to find clothes that fit but do it anyway, if you want the job. You don't need to be the best dressed for the job, just appropriately dressed for the position. It is unlikely that the boss will focus on your clothing as long as it is average and appropriate. Groom your face and hair, accessorize appropriately, and make sure that you are comfortable in the outfit and shoes you have chosen to wear.

There are plenty of obese people in all areas of the workforce. You may actually get that job or promotion before you have lost a significant amount of weight. While size does matter and people do judge you by your size (large or small), you can influence others by how you dress and groom yourself regardless of the size of your body.

When to Shop

On January 10, 2010 (weight 267; size 22/24), I finally got up the courage to walk into a Chico's Clothing Store. They are somewhat upscale and I was aware that I could not fit into the clothing sizes sold in the store. I had been shopping at the bookstore next door, was dressed casually, and on impulse,

I found myself walking right in the door. I took a breath and looked around. Not one sales person asked if they could help me and there were at least three of them standing around doing nothing. When thinner women came into the store, the sales people immediately offered to assist. I begin to look at the accessories, including the jewelry and scarves. Finally, a sales woman came over to help. She was the most poorly dressed and possibly couldn't afford to buy the clothing in the store for herself. I told her that I knew I could not fit into Chico's line of clothing but that I had lost 45 pounds and would eventually be able to shop there. I asked, "What is the largest size you carry?" She said they carried from size 2 to 16/18. I said thank you and purchased a lovely scarf. This took so much courage and I had to do it on a day when my self-esteem was at the top. I saw many beautiful clothes I would have loved to purchase. Someday, I will.

There are so many good reasons for going shopping for clothes, shoes, and accessories. Now that I have learned to shop, it has become much easier. Before I began this journey, I had allowed my wardrobe to become faded, stretched out, and pilled. Most of what I bought then was baggy because I thought "baggy" would hide my fat. There was no style; as long as it went around my body and had some room to spare, I bought it. I had lost all dignity. There are people who dislike shopping regardless of size and frequently that club includes men. Liking the task is not required. You may not have fun, at least not in the beginning. You are shopping to increase self-esteem, improve your personal appearance, and begin to open doors in your social and professional life.

Now about those good reasons for shopping: Walking around in the store is exercise. Believe it! You are *working out* when you're shopping, especially if you are large enough so that it is difficult for you to walk and move. Even if you are still in Plus Sizes, you can improve your wardrobe. And, *I repeat*, when you dress better, you feel better. When you feel better, you eat healthier. It is a cycle. Dress well; eat well. Dress badly; eat badly—probably unhealthy junk food. Therefore, shopping for clothes is part of maintaining that healthy, average size body, and feeling as though you belong in the world of the average.

With about every fifteen pounds lost, I found the need to replace pants and tops. Some clothes still fit me, but most started to look frumpy and sloppy at that point. When you are wearing clothes that fit, you feel better about yourself. Baggy clothes are a problem. They make you *feel* thinner than you are! However, they make you *look* heavier than you are. Wearing clothes that fit will encourage you in your journey to a healthy, average size body.

Good Riddance

It is important to get rid of clothes as they become too large for you. This is critical. You not only want to make space in your closet for the new clothes but you want to send a message to your brain that you won't be needing those large clothes ever again. Perhaps you cannot afford to go out and buy new clothes. Check out the Goodwill, garage sales, or discount stores. You might be surprised what you will find. Tailors can be expensive. Become friends with a sewing machine, if money is tight. If you never learned to sew, perhaps you know someone who could help you learn how to alter your clothes. Maybe a family member sews. Ask around. Many clothing items are easy to alter.

Finally, go shopping whether you plan to buy or not. If that feels too scary, try a little MicroStep. Just walk through a store and then go home. Do this for a few times and see if your courage for shopping increases. Walking through the store will both reduce your anxiety about shopping and is an opportunity for productive exercise. Whether you are only looking around or trying something on, the activity can keep you up to date as to what is available and what size you are wearing. While you are at it, greet some of your fellow shoppers. This will help you feel as if you belong. Most likely, the other person will smile and offer a greeting in return. It never hurts to add a little social exercise to the task. While you are in the store, you might find a special item on sale and buy it. It might help you feel better about how you are dressing.

Learning to dress better is hard work. Part of that work is becoming familiar with the stores in your area. It is helpful to know what they carry and what works for you in each store. For many obese people, just going into a clothing store creates severe anxiety. As I stated, walking through the stores when you are not planning to buy something is one way to help you get beyond the dread and anxiety of shopping.

Men, I do not want to see your eyes glazing over at the idea of shopping. Everything I'm saying about shopping applies to you, too. Macho men do shop! Walking though a store and looking around is exercise for you as well. Some men like to take their partner, wife, or girlfriend along. If that helps, then by all means, do it. You do not have to stay in the store for hours. For your first shopping trip, perhaps you just stay five minutes and glance at a couple of items. We are talking about MicroSteps—and all it takes is one at a time.

Learning from TV's "What Not to Wear"

As I've mentioned in earlier chapters, I loved the television show on The Learning Channel called *What Not to Wear*. The new episodes have ended but there are still reruns airing. The show had two stylists (Stacy London and Clinton Kelly) who would surprise a badly dressed person with a trip to New York City and $5,000 to purchase a new wardrobe. The catch was that the person had to allow the stylists to throw away his or her old unflattering wardrobe. The stylists would teach the person how dress for their body type and lifestyle. The stylists taught the person how to shop, helped the person shop, and then got to approve the new $5,000 wardrobe.

When I first started to watch this show, I found the stylists a bit arrogant and annoying. I stayed with it because I knew how badly I was dressing. I had been living in a small town for a few years and felt completely out of touch with the trends and styles. I knew I needed help. Once I started watching it, I could not stop. I watched it almost daily until I felt I had a clear sense of what was fashionable and stylish. I knew it would take me a while to be able to buy those clothes and look good but at least I had the knowledge in my head. That was my first shopping MicroStep.

As I began to go shopping with a little more confidence, I began to have a better eye for what would look best on my body type. I also discovered some things about how to put an outfit together that I had not known before. When I was younger and smaller, I thought I was dressing well but *What Not to Wear* taught me more about how to be stylish than I had ever known in the past. Here are a few of the things I learned:

- Being stylish and fashionable is hard work.
- Most people, even those with average size bodies, struggle to find things that fit perfectly.
- Get rid of clothes that are too large, too small, or don't look good on you.
- Keep shopping until you find something that fits and works.
- Do not put things together that are too "matchy matchy." That means do not buy pink pants, a pink blouse, pink shoes, pink hat, and a pink purse. They need to go together, not match.
- Combine one item that has color and pair it with neutrals. That is more stylish and you will look as though you know what you are doing.
- Dress your age. Do not dress as though you're competing with teenagers or as though you're older than you are.
- If it does not fit, do not wear it. Without fit, there is no fashion.
- Some things go with other things (i.e. too dressy for a day shoe, too casual for an evening shoe). For example, men you don't wear sandals with a dress suit.
- Straight leg pants are good for most people.
- If something does not fit, try something else.
- Do not buy pants that are pleated; they make your stomach look bigger.
- If you cannot afford a tailor, learn to sew.
- Women, an hourglass shape is good at any size.
- Men, a jacket will help disguise the size of a stomach.
- Go shopping more often. Don't wait until you are wearing rags or looking horrible.

When you are shopping and the clothes are not fitting, don't get discouraged. They will fit eventually. Just stay with it long enough to try on a few outfits and then stop for the day. Go buy something else, such as make-up, jewelry, new after-shave, or shoes. They are easier to find in the right size. Okay, I did not get that from *What Not to Wear*, I made that one up, and it helps.

Since I began the journey of the HRRTs, my jewelry wardrobe has improved tremendously. In the beginning, it was too frustrating to shop for clothes. I would shop for an hour and get discouraged. Rather than going home empty-handed I'd stop by the jewelry counter or accessories section, buy a little something, and then I would feel better. I had something to show for my effort and time spent. I was still improving my physical presentation and building my self-esteem. Eventually, as I applied what I had learned from *What Not to Wear* about how to shop for my body type, the clothes began to fit. In the meantime, I had increased my purse, shoe, and jewelry wardrobe.

Accepting Your Body

The human body does not come retouched, blemish-free, with digital liposuction, magically smoothed out wrinkles, or hips that shrink with the click of a mouse. That only happens for models on the covers of magazines. It is not real so let's get over it and look at our bodies as a work of art created by a master designer. For example, an old minister friend had a favorite expression, "God don't make no junk." We need to find the beauty in the work of art that is our body.

I'm sure you are thinking that a flabby stomach is not much of a work of art. I understand; that is how I felt at 315 pounds.

Since we also know, but seem to forget, that there is no such thing as perfection, we must learn to accept *good enough* without compromising too much.

When I was shopping in the only two stores in town that carried my size, it was much more difficult to accept my body and try to dress fashionably. I was unable to find a store that carried stylish, quality clothes in my size when I was 2X, 3X, or 4X. That made it harder to accept my body; however, I worked towards that goal by acknowledging the beauty in my face, my eyes, and my hair.

Everyone has some part of his or her body that is attractive, if you are willing to look and you can give up the notion of perfection. Most of us had to give up long ago the notion that we had the world's most intelligent brain or the world's biggest bank account. Letting go of the notion that we need to have the perfect body is difficult but just as realistic.

Keeping a Shopping Journal

In the beginning, my shopping trips were depressing, physically challenging, and emotionally draining. Looking at my journal from those earlier days, I remember how fragile I felt and how difficult were those first shopping MicroSteps. I started to try to improve my wardrobe long before I had even lost a pound. In the beginning, it seemed impossible to look better. For months, the only things that improved were my shoe and earring collections. Even that helped my confidence.

One day, I walked into a regular department store and began to look around for the Plus Size clothes. I saw the Petites, Junior, and Regular Size clothes right away. They were well-displayed and well-organized, but the Plus Size area was hidden away in a back corner, which was crowded, and messy. There were no displays, and many items were falling off the hangers. It did not look anything like the beautiful shops I had been watching on *What Not to Wear*.

Keeping in mind the things I had learned, I decided to ignore the mess and start looking for things that might fit. I was still a Plus Size 3X and that is generally an easy size to find in the Plus Size section of the store. I found a few tops and a couple of pants that I thought were *good enough*. I say *good enough* because they were not made of nice fabrics and the pants had elastic waists. There were no chic clothes in my size and I had to settle for what I could get but at least they were new. I made sure the colors were nice for my skin tone and purchased the new tops and pants. I was not getting what I wanted but I still felt I was moving forward.

Months later, I bought some pants that had zippers and buttons. I had finally graduated out of pants with elastic waists. At the same time, I also found a couple of tops made of nicer fabrics. Since I still hadn't found a good tailor, I spent the next day altering a couple of tops and hemming the new pants.

Yes, it's harder for me to keep clothes fitting when I keep changing sizes, but I am not complaining. For a while every three, six, or eight months nothing fit again, and so I would have to donate the too large clothes and buy new ones. Some things are easy to tailor; I actually enjoy sewing now and then.

One day I hemmed a pair of beautiful dark gray pants. I did not notice but my pinking shears cut a one-inch hole in the front of the left leg just above the bottom of the hem. As I was finishing the last of the hem, I saw the inch long cut. Upset, I tried to fix it without success. The hole was too large and my efforts to repair it just made it worse. I threw them away; I'd have to replace them. I tried not to let it ruin my day. I forced myself to get on with my weekend. I found a good movie to watch and drowned my sorrows in a sad love gone wrong story. At least, I did not go for ice cream.

A month later, I went into the same store where I had purchased the pants and looked for the beautiful dark gray pants. They did not have my size, at that time a 22. I decided to try the size 20 and to my amazement and delight, they fit. As it turned out, the pants I ruined would have been too large in a month and I would have had to replace them anyway. What a lesson! Drink that lemonade!

After losing some more weight, I once again found that my pants were all but falling off my body. I had to go shopping again. I found some white pants in size 20. They fit! The grey pants fitting in size 20 was not a quirk after all! I had started out as a size 28/30 pant size. This was thrilling. I did not buy them because I felt the fabric was not flattering; it was too thin. I did buy some navy pants and a top. More and more, I was beginning to find things that fit. Instead of just buying something in a rush, I was now able to spend time deciding if the item flattered my figure, my coloring, and went with my lifestyle. What a thrill to be able to buy clothes that look good on me and not just buy what goes around my enormous body.

Again, it is work to keep up with one's changing body. Whenever I lose another fifteen pounds, it's not always convenient to drop everything and go shopping again. I work forty hours a week and don't have much time for shopping sprees. Moreover, replacing the majority of your clothes every six to eight months gets expensive—especially when I know the new things will need to be replaced before they wear out. I try to keep it simple by buying half a dozen work pants, two pairs of jeans, and ten or so tops. That way I am not investing in a major wardrobe every few months, but am able to look my best for work and casual times. At this point, I am not buying the most expensive clothing and I am not buying investment pieces. That time is coming.

It has been years since I wore skirts and dresses. Recently, I crossed that bridge and decided to shop for some more feminine items and dressier outfits. I admit it felt a little scary to think about doing this because back when I was wearing dresses and skirts people wore stockings. Today, it's the fashion to go bare legged, wear tights, or wear only certain colors of stockings. Intimidating!

There is so much to figure out and so many adjustments to make on this journey. Reflecting back on how far I have come helps. My goal is to present myself as a healthy, average size person who just happens to dress stylishly. It is a dream that seems to get closer each day.

I am excited about the shopping adventures ahead and try to keep informed as to the current trends. Being aware of the styles does not mean you have to buy them. For me, that awareness and knowing how to shop is a big confidence booster. I truly hope it is for you, too.

To put it simply, when you look your best, you feel more confident, and are more likely to move forward in your life. When you are moving forward in your life, you are not setting on the sofa—wasting your life as a *couch potato*.

Now, get up, get dressed, and get going!

CHAPTER 11

Sagging Skin and Wrinkles

FACING YOUR FEARS IS NEVER EASY. For several years, I avoided losing weight because I was over fifty and thought significant weight loss would result in sagging skin around my stomach and upper legs, an older looking face, and floppy arms. While I was severely obese, I loved having people tell me I looked ten or fifteen years younger than my real age. To say the least, I was imagining the worst. Losing weight slowly, in MicroSteps, has resulted in allowing my skin to shrink and I am not nearly as saggy as I feared I would be. People continue to tell me I look ten years younger than my real age.

As I got larger and larger, I felt increasingly uncomfortable with the pain of trying to walk. I was humiliated by being unable to find stylish clothes that fit and overcome with shame for allowing my body to get so large. I finally decided the sagging skin might be better than my current state of obesity. After all, you can put stylish clothing over sagging skin. Only your lovers and doctors need know the truth. While I doubt that I will ever be interested, there is also the option of plastic surgery.

Consider Your Options

Often in life, we do not have perfect choices and must cope with the reality of the situation in which we find ourselves. For example, a thirteen-year-old girl finds herself pregnant. Let's face it, she has choices; however, none of them is perfect for a thirteen-year-old girl. She could have the baby and keep it, give it up for adoption, let her parents or someone else raise it, or have an abortion. Regardless of your belief system, none of these choices is perfect for a thirteen-year-old girl. We could spend days talking about how she got into the situation or how she was a victim of a smooth-talking boy; in the end, the choices left to her are not perfect and she must cope with the reality of her pregnancy.

Once you find yourself overweight, that is the reality of your life, and your choices are limited and challenging. If you stay large and get larger, your health is at risk. Your self-esteem may prevent you from enjoying relationships and work success. There are so many reasons to decide to take the journey of the HRRTs to achieve a healthy, average size body.

While you may still be small enough that after you lose the weight your skin will shrink and look tight, those who are larger may need to grieve the loss of that tight, young looking skin. It may have been easier for me because I was over fifty when I finally decided to take this journey to a healthy, average size body. After realizing I was going to get old anyway, I accepted that we all eventually get some sagging skin. I am not sure how I would have felt if I had been years younger and needed to compete in the world of youth.

Choosing to end the stress of weight issues for the last time is not about going on a diet. It is about changing your lifestyle by changing your Habits, Routines, Rituals, and Traditions. This not only has a major impact on you; it will affect the lives of those around you. In the end, it is not only about choosing to accept sagging skin but it is also about being willing to confront the negative HRRTs that have gotten you into this situation in the first place. Habits, Routines, Rituals, and Traditions are not only yours personally; you share them with your spouse or partner, your children, your extended family, and your friends.

I remember seeing a friend lose weight and experiencing a feeling of loss because I had been so used to her the way she was. When she lost weight, her personality changed; she developed new and different interests. Suddenly, there were no more long lunches overeating and talking about all the thin people walking by. In the past we'd assume they were snobs and must have attitude issues. It made us feel better. We also assumed they were laughing at us because we were fat. We ended up spending less time together. While it might have happened anyway, I think it was in part because we lost our shared interest of overeating. I did not have the confidence to join her on ski trips, outings to the beach, travel opportunities that required airplane travel (and seats I couldn't fit into comfortably), or at the nicer restaurants. My weight was in the way. You may find that as you lose the weight, your family and friends need to go through an adjustment period to discover how to be with the new you. My family was used to my sitting home, watching television, and cooking fattening holiday meals. They hardly knew what to do when I decided to ditch the fattening Easter Lunch and serve a healthier meal with plenty of fresh salad and vegetables.

Suddenly, I was off the sofa and doing things out in the community. My style and interests changed as my confidence changed. I also lost the desire to be with people who only wanted to indulge in overeating and watching television. People who had expected me to be a certain way needed time to figure out how to be with the new me. Perhaps, I should have said the *real me* is not a person sitting in shame in the corner of my life due to obesity. Give friends and family time. Help them take MicroSteps so they may get to know the way you are now. Help them understand that this is the real you, the one that you have been hiding beneath the weight. Do not allow others who miss the larger you prevent or interfere with your decision to achieve and keep that healthy, average size body.

Transcending the Trauma of Obesity

How does one make such a decision to stop overeating? For me, it was about being sick and tired of the physical pain of trying to walk, not fitting into chairs, and knowing that I was living far below my potential because of the trauma of my obesity. Obesity is not a trauma in the traditional sense. It is, however, traumatic to live daily for years on end knowing that people are looking at you and thinking about how large you are. It feels traumatic to be too large to sit in an airplane seat, not to be able to wear fashionable clothing, and to be unable to walk up a flight of stairs without losing your breath. It feels traumatic to eat a meal in a restaurant and wish people were not looking at you, because you know they are thinking about the fat girl eating those ribs and fries. Yet, I still ate the ribs and fries and just tolerated the shame. Living in shame is horrible.

After losing forty pounds, I began to see that the fears of having severely sagging skin were more in my mind than in reality. It was a nice surprise to see that my face did not look as old as I had thought it would. Part of my waist was coming back and without the sagging skin. I was still waiting to see what would happen to that part of my stomach where I had gotten exceptionally large. By this time, it did not matter if it sagged. The loss of forty pounds had already given me more energy and I was feeling better about my appearance and myself.

One thing that helped was looking at other people's skin. Most of us do not really look at each other. We sort of look at what another person wears but we do not look at each other's body to see shape and size. I began to look at other people, subtly so as not to appear to stare. I got the idea from watching *What Not to Wear* on The Learning Channel. The stylists, Stacy London and Clinton Kelly, really looked at the contributors' (the guests') bodies. After discussing the contributor's body type, they'd point out how their clothes fit and how they could choose clothes that were more flattering. It helped me to realize that most people did not have perfect bodies in the first place. I generalized that insight to the streets and into my life. I saw many different body types, ages of people, and noticed that most people have something they do not like about their bodies, something that sags, and are aging in one way or another. Some of the people I'd always thought were the most beautiful, before I looked more closely, had sagging arms or winkles in their faces. I still think they are beautiful. When I really looked, other people were not always wearing clothes that fit perfectly or were of great quality, or flattered their body types any better than my clothes flattered mine. I stopped looking only at the beautiful actors and models and started looking at every-day folks. It helped. I discovered that being average was not a bad thing and that became my goal.

Loss-Benefits Ratio

After losing forty-five pounds, I discovered to my great happiness that I was able to shop in stores that do not carry plus sizes. Now, that does not mean that everything in those stores fit me but I was able to find some pants, some tops, and enjoyed just being able to go into a dressing room and find things were large enough to zip and button. For the first time in many years, I was able to choose what actually looked good on me and not just buy something because it would cover my enormous shape. This was a wonderful moment and increased my motivation immeasurably.

I was still around ninety pounds from being an average size. I still had a stomach that hung over as if I'd been pregnant. Yes, I continued to be concerned about what my skin would look like at the end; however, this moment helped me realize that regardless of what my skin did, it was worth it. I loved being able to choose stylish clothes. Getting rid of those negative HRRTs was no loss at all considering the payoff.

Years ago, I had minor knee surgery. For a long time, every step hurt and I thought it was all because of my bad knees. After losing fifty, then sixty, pounds, I discovered that my knees were not so bad after all. Yes, they still have arthritis; however, I can walk without pain and with tremendous energy on most days. What a joy! I will take a little sagging skin over bad knees any day.

The truth: Human beings do lose their shape, skin eventually sags, and we get age spots on our hands. Only diamonds retain their shape forever. I am reminded of the words from the musical "Diamonds Are a Girl's Best Friend", *Square-cut or pear-shaped these rocks don't lose their shape...* I am all about reality; I would rather be a little saggy but able to live my life in dignity and without pain.

Sagging skin will never stop me from living my life; obesity robbed me of the ability to take pleasure in a social life, enjoy daily tasks, and limited my career opportunities. Yes, give me a little sagging skin any day. I have my life back!

PART THREE

Life Among the Average Size

CHAPTER 12

Living in the Mainstream

FOR SOMEONE WHO HAS LOST an enormous amount of weight in just a few short months, perhaps as a result going on a starvation diet or having bariatric surgery, the dramatic physical changes to the body can be unsettling, especially when they look in the mirror or get feedback from family and friends. As much as being thin was their goal, this kind of abrupt change can create anxiety, as we discussed in the beginning of our journey together.

However, since you and I have been on a *slow lifestyle change* as the result of losing weight in MicroSteps instead of doing it rapidly, we are not burdened with the shock of suddenly being thin and not knowing how to be happy with the results. We have enjoyed the slow-but-steady changes to our bodies over many months, if not years. We now feel the pride and comfort of joining in on those daily activities that average size people all around us seem to do without thought. No longer are we on a life raft in the middle of the ocean crying, "Water water everywhere and not a drop to drink."

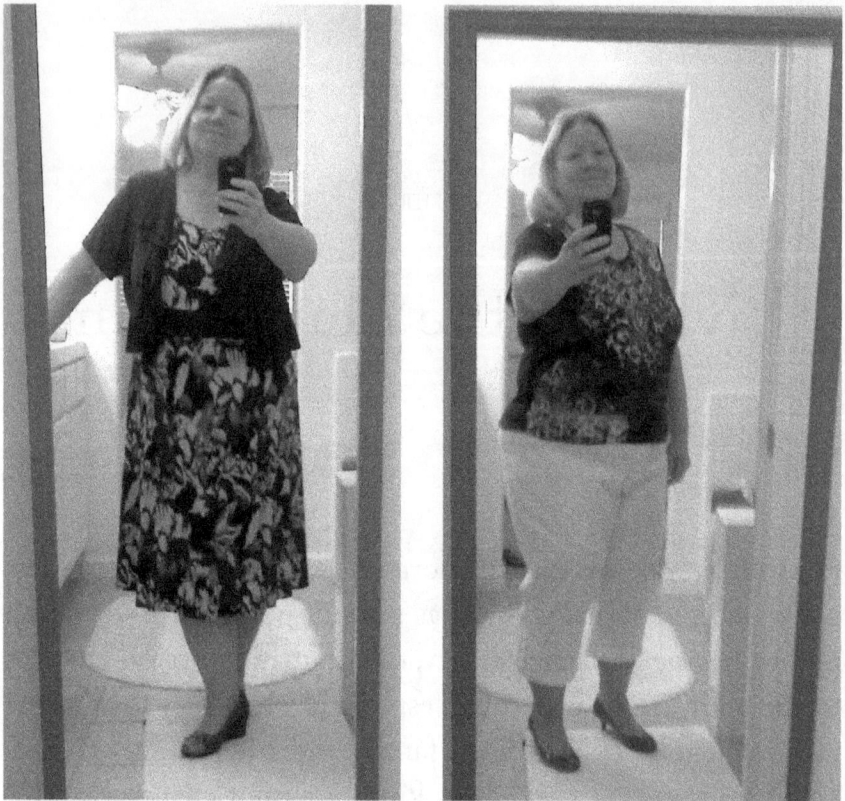

December 2014, Weight 234 lbs. What to wear? It was difficult trying to wrap my head around the changes.

Unless you've been living on an island and no one has seen you since you started your MicroSteps journey, there is no *big moment* when suddenly everyone notices your weight loss as you make your grand entrance—in *your new thin body*—at a gathering of family and friends. You know, the moment when suddenly everyone notices that you are half your size! Because of making changes in MicroSteps, your family and friends will have been in your day-to-day life as your body slowly changed. Your spouse or lover has made love to you at your largest and every size in-between. There is no sudden shock of change.

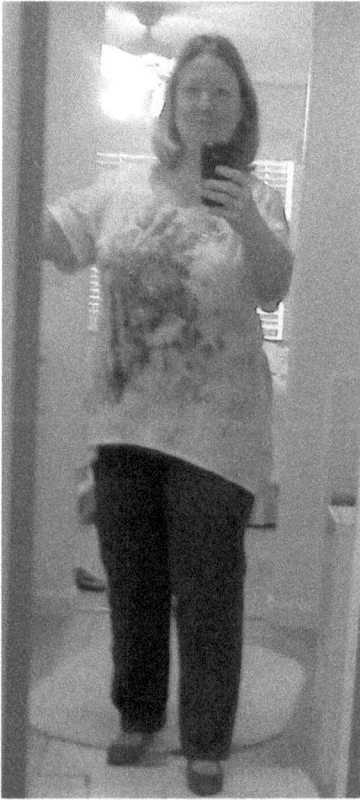

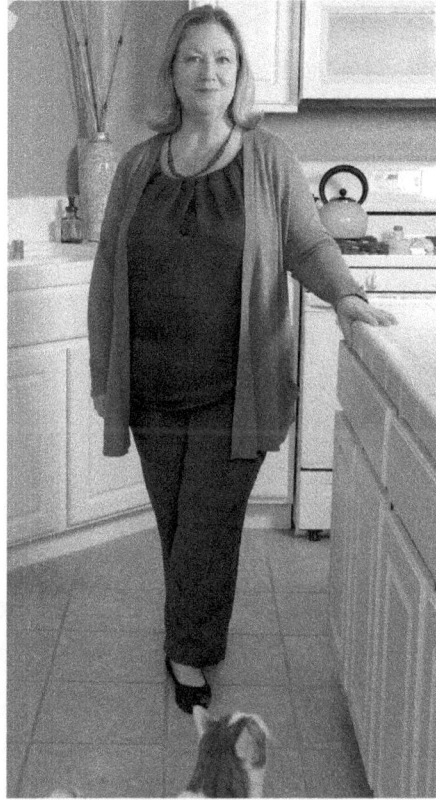

December 2014, Weight 234 lbs. More to lose but feeling healthy and average. Oliver photo bombs. Guess he's impressed too!

A Dream Come True

My experience has been that those people closest to me did not say much. They were with me daily or almost daily. The weight loss was so slow that they adjusted along with me as it was happening. My family and friends who live out of town were the only ones to notice with that *WOW* reaction, which I was okay with, but it did not mean as much as having someone experience me as an ordinary size on a daily basis. Living life among the average, being lost in the mainstream, with my weight *not* being an issue, has been my greatest reward—a *dream come true*. I just wanted to be an average size person and finally I was. If you are obese, you understand. You also know the joy that bubbles up inside your soul when you find that you can walk through a turnstile at an amusement park, sit on an airplane seat, wear a beautiful dress from a mainstream store, or simply take a walk with your partner. Your spouse, children, best friend, and the others in your day-to-day life may now take your size for granted. When my people began to see me as just another person, I was delighted. I love that! The joy is in the small things that only those who have lived large may ever truly know.

For the first half of my life, I was an average size. If I had been obese all those years, I suppose I would have still felt obese after my body had again become an average size, a common disconnect for many people who lose a lot of weight. My own experience has been the opposite. While I was obese, I kept bumping into furniture and trying to squeeze into spaces that were too small for me. Now that I am nearing average size again, I feel that I have come home. I am able to move about more easily and feel more like myself, although there are some occasions when I am pleasantly surprised that I fit into a booth at a restaurant, can wear an article of clothing that looks too small, or still have energy after climbing a flight of stairs.

It is so much easier to give myself a pedicure now that my stomach is not preventing me from touching my toes. I used to struggle to keep my toenails trimmed and now I am able to go ahead and polish them, if I choose. I know many people get professional pedicures; however, I always seem to find something else I would rather do.

Determining your goal weight can be a challenge. I wanted my weight to be low enough to keep my body healthy but high enough so that I would not have to sacrifice too much in an effort to be *thin*. I knew if my target weight was too low that I could end up discouraged and possibly fail to stick with it. I considered my age, my lifestyle, and my health in making this all-important decision. Since being thin was not my objective in the first place, I often remind myself that I am not in *show business*, I do not need to *walk a catwalk*, and I have no *photo shoots*. This helps. Accepting *good enough* is the first step. Remembering that when my weight was 315 pounds all I wanted was to be average. That helps, too. I am nearing average now and I choose to rejoice instead of continuing to seek a smaller size body.

All I know is that I never want to weigh 315 pounds again. Being that large was miserable. I fear going back so much that even the normal, daily weight fluctuations scare me. Having healthy new HRRTs to rely on does not necessarily eliminate the anxious thoughts about regaining the weight—memories of those obese years die hard.

Keeping Your Eye on the HRRTs

My concerns about regaining weight nudges me to keep looking at the Habits, Routines, Rituals, and Traditions that caused me to become obese in the first place and that is good. You may be thinking, "Isn't this what we did at the beginning of this journey?" You are correct. We have already faced the negative HRRTs and slowly, via MicroSteps, changed the ones that were preventing a healthy, average size body. During that process, we looked at the HRRTs that were interfering with weight loss and were, in one way or another, related directly to food.

In order to find balance in life so that you obtain and maintain your target weight, it is now time to become more aware of the Habits, Routines, Rituals, and Traditions that are in other areas of your life as well. These areas include physical health, spiritual, romance, family, financial, social life, work, career, education, and day-to-day activities. If you don't keep these parts of your life in balance, the HRRTs can and will sneak in and sabotage your eating.

When my life is out of balance, I feel like a ship that is rocking on a rough sea. I'm in danger and I know it. Before long, I am running like crazy back to those old HRRTs for comfort. So it is wise for me to identify my weak spots ahead of time. Since a chain, as they say, is only as strong as its weakest link, then one little negative HRRT can do a whole boatload of damage. My weakest links are sour dough bread with butter, tortilla chips, cheese, and desserts. I also hate to exercise. However, as much as I hate giving up daily sour dough bread with butter, tortilla chips, cheese, and desserts, I hate obesity more.

I manage my weak spots by continuing to work on negative MicroSteps. Each night, when it feels like snack time, I find myself thinking that it is no big deal to have just one small ____. (You fill in the blank.) It is tempting to tell myself that I am only having this little treat once and nothing is off limits in the journey of the HRRTs. It took me a while but I finally realized that my mind was playing a trick on me. That nightly little snack was the birth of a new negative Habit trying to have its way with me.

Balancing the exceptions to healthy eating is a big challenge. I eat whatever I want, whenever I want. Most of the time, I realize that my wants have changed and that my desires may be trusted, but not always. One way to recognize that there is a problem is to pay attention to how often you are eating something that in the past was supporting the obesity. We easily create Routines and the frequency you eat something will be a major clue for monitoring your HRRTs. Remember, your wants must support the reality of maintaining that healthy, average size body.

Don't get scared. By now, you know how to identify a negative HRRT, choose the easiest possible goal, and move forward in MicroSteps. We human beings are complex creatures and it is difficult to keep life managed. Not to worry, your new HRRTs will not be derailed so easily. Still, it is risky to allow things to get too out of balance just because you have stopped paying attention to them. They are like children. We need to keep an eye on them or they will stray from our expectations.

Living a Life in Balance

Some basic areas of stress are challenging for most people. These areas may include finances, health, relationships with others, and the general daily tasks of life. There are also others and I am sure you can list them without even thinking very hard. Now that you have achieved, or are close to achieving, a healthy, average size body, it is time to look carefully at any HRRTs that may still be preventing healthy living in some area of your life.

Where do you find you are still the most stressed? That might be a good starting place. For example, are you worried about money on a daily basis? Are your children having problems in school? Is your marriage unhappy? Do you need

210 / The End of Living Large

to make a career change? Are you having spiritual questions, romance problems, or education difficulties? This is an individual decision and you might need to do some prioritizing in order to determine the best place to begin.

To assure success, choose one of the easier areas and identify a simple goal. Next, choose one tiny MicroStep you could take to begin to reach that goal. Slowly, in MicroSteps, work on that goal to help you to change the Habit, Routine, Ritual, or Tradition that is causing stress or making your life out of balance. Do you remember the discussion in Chapter 2 on *Attending to Your Basic Needs*? Well, we are simply taking this to the next level. We do this because managing stress is a critical part of managing weight.

Initially, trying to manage the stressors that cause life to get out of balance may cause you to feel overwhelmed, even panicky, which can lead you to feeling like a failure. Don't give up. Continue to identify the areas of your life that are causing disruption. Choose the ones that you would like to work on. By now, you know the drill. Simply take one MicroStep after another until you have reached your goal and change has occurred. Little by little, you will begin to experience a healthier balance in your life. It is easier to manage your weight when your life feels managed as well.

Family and Social Relationships

For many people, the biggest stressor in life is that of relationships with others. In weight management, this is certainly a big issue. While other stressors can be equally as challenging, I would like to spend a little extra time right now talking about relationships with others and the challenge of keeping that area of life in balance. You must have managed some of those issues to get to this point in your journey, but the challenge of relationships is unending, even those most dear.

Ask yourself about the people in your life: Who is supportive? Who builds your self-esteem? Who drags you down? Who eats badly or encourages you to stay home on the sofa? Who stimulates your creative spirit and makes you want to do more? Whom do you most enjoy?

Now ask the more difficult questions: Is there someone in your life who hurts you mentally or physically, drags you down when you are with them, or causes you to feel badly about yourself? Identify the people are who are negatively influencing your Habits, Routines, Rituals, and Traditions and consider limiting your time with them or avoiding them altogether.

In my obese days, I spent my free time on the sofa watching television. It took a little doing to develop new Routines and make sure they were healthy ones. I needed to find other people who were interested in getting out and doing things. Doing an activity alone was not fulfilling enough. These social activities needed to be ones that supported a healthy lifestyle. I needed to share my social time with people who understood this, who were healthy or striving to become healthy, who were a good influence, and not with people who were a negative or toxic influence.

What do you do about those friends and family members who are not supportive or have unhealthy lifestyles themselves? Naturally, you don't want to dump family or dear friends, unless they're physically or emotionally abusive; however, you have to start thinking of people who are not supportive in the same way you think of foods that aren't good for you. You indulge in them occasionally but not as a regular diet. I eat cake, ice cream, and candy occasionally, but that is not part of my daily Habits, Routines, or Rituals. I try to reserve those tasty desserts for special occasions such as a Traditional holiday event. Similarly, you may decide to interact with someone, perhaps for business reasons, but then free yourself of them as quickly as possible. The people I choose to spend most of my time with need to be supportive of my healthy living. The risk is simply too great to do otherwise.

The Sabotage Club

Let's discuss the members of the Sabotage Club. They are the folks in your life who love you so much they want to feed you their special homemade desserts, family dinners of pot roasts with potatoes and lots of gravy, share a pizza and beer with you, insist on going out for ribs and fries, and they will not take no for an answer. There is also the special Gift Givers Committee of this club. You know who they are. They bring wrapped gifts of muffins to you at work, or buy you boxes of chocolates, and give you cookies. Of course, by now, you know that some of their behaviors are coming out of deeply embedded Traditions and Rituals from their own lives. That is fine but you still need to know how to manage these situations, especially those members of the Club who are Specialists in Guilt Trips and Hurt Feelings.

For me, the difficult part is not in saying no to someone who is offering me a fabulous dessert or deliciously fattening meal. I try to be polite and graciously decline without hurting his or her feelings. If I choose, I can eat one indulgent meal without causing a weight management problem. I try not to schedule too many events where I know this will be an issue. Instead, I offer to do the cooking myself, take the person out to eat, or to go to a movie.

My biggest challenge is deciding what to do with that kindly gifted box of chocolates or basket of my favorite muffins from someone trying to show their love. If I keep it, I will eat it. If I don't take it home, I will think about it and then buy something like it to eat. Most of the time, I eat one or two and get rid of the rest. I know this may sound horrible, but I put the rest in a trash container that is exceptionally dirty and disgusting. That way the nasty trashcan in which I last saw my goodies blemishes my memory of them and they are temptations no more. I will tell the person who gave them to me that they were delicious; I ate a couple, and the rest undoubtedly were delicious. I say thank you and move on. Sometimes I have a little sidebar with my friend, explain that the treats are just too tasty, and request that she or he not bring me any more such temptations.

If you find you are unable to be honest with the members in your Sabotage Club, you might need to find a therapist and process this a bit. This is especially true if your spouse or partner happens to be the President of the Club. As long as you have been kind and polite, you are not responsible for the hurt feelings of other people. This is their issue and fixing them is not your job. Your job is to live your life as a healthy, average size person. Most of your family and friends will come to understand. Those who do not may have deeper problems and eating their unhealthy foods is not the way to help them.

When it comes to eating in a healthy manner and taking care of your healthy, average size body, it is okay for it to be *all about you*.

Physical and Mental Activities

Getting life in balance and managing the stressors is not the only challenge. You cannot maintain a physically healthy lifestyle without participating in the mainstream of life. As I have said before, this includes social, physical, mental, and spiritual involvement. I repeat this because it is so important and something that the extremely obese find challenging. Years of living life in an obese condition puts a dent in your self-esteem. Even after losing the weight, you may not feel as though you belong in the mainstream of life. It's as if you don't believe *you deserve* that *white picket fence*. Well, you do so grab a brush and let's get painting!

Our bodies need to move in order to use up the calories we take in and even though we do not count calories, moving your body must be something you do daily. There is a big payoff for simply doing the basics such as keeping the house clean, planning and cooking meals, shopping, gardening, playing outside with your children, taking classes, joining a sports team, and simply spending time out and about.

Exercising is hard to accept. I work hard long hours. I am exhausted at night. I have minimal time during the day to exercise. Weekends get lost amongst the chores, housecleaning, bill paying, family obligations, and trying to find time for a social life. My struggle to manage physical activity is the same struggle that caused the 315 pounds in the first place. The answer is in the MicroSteps and keeping life in balance. I never said it would be easy; however, it is doable.

My inner adolescent wants the world to believe that I have succeeded and that I am perfect. It does not want to admit that other people have good ideas or might be right about exercising. My adolescent holds to the belief that, "I can do this without exercising, thank you!" My inner adolescent also hates to feel pressured and wants respect. All it takes is one person suggesting that I join a gym and I am on the sofa for weeks. Do you have a rebellious inner adolescent? I suspect we all do.

I often ponder: Do I allow this inner teenager to prevent me from exercise and trigger a return to 315 pounds? That is the choice. The task is to weigh the consequences of this decision. It is far too easy to allow my inner adolescent to rule my life and sabotage my healthy, average size body. It is a war and my weapon is the MicroSteps that helped me lose weight in the first place.

When I get home from work in the evening, there are usually a few neighbors standing around outside chatting. Even though I am exhausted and only want to hit that sofa for the night, I try to spend a little time with them. This is good because I am walking, standing, and enjoying their company. I know that I am not burning hundreds of calories this way, but I always feel a little more energized after those few minutes of socialization.

You may need to begin in MicroSteps to get yourself going. That is okay. As long as you do something socially or physically you are moving forward and can maintain life as a healthy, average size person. Average size people move and interact with others.

While I have focused on the physical and social more than the mental, it is important to remember mental exercise is a critical part of getting and keeping life in balance. It is necessary to continue to gain knowledge as a way of life. As you settle into the mainstream of life as a healthy, average size person, try learning something new on a regular basis. The act of regularly gaining knowledge can be a wonderful new Habit or Routine.

There are many different ways to gain knowledge such as reading a book, going to a lecture, learning things off the Web, Food Network, or Learning Channel, and seeking out new information for personal growth. These are all good ways to gain knowledge. In my own case, I always like a little variety in how I learn things, just as I like a little variety in my food choices.

When I am watching a cooking show, sometimes I just sit back and enjoy it. Other times I write down a recipe for later use. Still another day I may look up the recipe online, go into the kitchen, and get cooking.

What you put into your mind is what will come out in actions, behaviors, and beliefs. Put in knowledge about healthy relationships, finances, nutrition, or fashion and trust that it will come out in a delightful and positive way. It does take time but that is how *THE END OF LIVING LARGE* works.

General Self-discipline

You would think that all there is to living with your hard-earned healthy, average size body is to keep on eating in the healthy manner established by the new HRRTs and enjoy it. I thought so too, at first. However, because I had so much more physical and mental energy, I wanted to do more than that. You would be surprised how an occasional movie, going out to dinner, spending an evening at a local concert, or just reading a book can add to your life. The good news was that I was up, out, and moving. The bad news was that I was finding it more difficult to go to bed in time to get those seven to eight hours of sleep.

When I first started losing weight, I became a bit of a social butterfly. Suddenly, I was calling people to go to lunch, spending more time shopping, standing outside visiting with the neighbors, volunteering in professional organizations. I was getting out of the house and looking for things to do. Before I knew it, I had myself so busy that I was starting to feel overwhelmed, beginning to eat on the run, snacking to keep up my energy, and sabotaging my new healthy HRRTs.

It soon became clear to me that self-discipline was required if I wanted to live my life as a healthy, average size person. This helps nurture your new HRRTs as they change naturally over time. They need tender guidance to make sure they continue to support your new healthier body. Just because you have the energy to go to that concert on a weeknight, knowing you have to get up at five o'clock the next morning for a work, does not mean you should allow yourself to go. It is important to get enough rest each day. If not, you will find it harder to avoid snacking as a means of replenishing the energy to make up for the lack of sleep.

Keep your kitchen stocked with easy to prepare healthy food choices so you can nurture your new HRRTs. As you begin to get out and socialize more, you'll find that your food life requires more planning or you'll end up grabbing whatever is quick, perhaps fast food, and not eating healthy meals. Keeping the kitchen stocked with healthy, easy-to-prepare choices helps at the end of a long workday, after a social outing, when family schedules are demanding, or when you do not feel like making dinner a major event.

When I have a day at home or do not feel like going out, I love to cook. I may put on a big pot of chili, bake a casserole, stovetop grill fifteen or twenty boneless chicken breasts, or make my favorite chicken tortilla soup. I then enjoy a healthy meal and freeze the rest in individual servings. That way I have some healthy choices on those days when I do not feel like cooking or my schedule is too demanding. Cooking on a day at home also prevents me from just sitting and watching television. At least, I am up and down as the food demands my attention. Cooking keeps me off the sofa, sends me out to the grocery store for some exercise, and uses calories as I stand to prepare the food. In addition, it gives me a sense of being in control and a satisfaction that I am helping to maintain my healthy, average size body.

Deferred Gratification

Part of living life as a healthy, average size person is going shopping for new clothes as a Routine to make sure you always look your best. While there are many good reasons to keep your wardrobe stylish and size appropriate, again, balance is called for. Obviously, it is not okay to become so indulgent with shopping that you get yourself into debt or financial difficulty. No one needs a new addiction: Shopping needs to be something that is helpful but not something from which you have to recover! Similarly, developing a healthy social life is not about going out every night, getting drunk, and neglecting work or family responsibilities. Again, balance is the key. Deferring gratification is simply learning to say no and using a little self-discipline in order to maintain a healthy way of life.

You are Already Maintaining

If you have traveled the journey described in this book, you have spent a long time changing your HRRTs. The magic of this journey is in its slowness. It is such a slow journey that you have already been maintaining your healthy, average size body without realizing it. Your lifestyle has changed. Believe it! By the time you achieve your healthy, average size body you will have been eating the right way for a year or more. Your new Habits have become a part of you. Managing those Habits, Rituals, and Traditions is ongoing, if you want to remain a healthy, average size person. Our HRRTs keep on changing as our lives, chronological ages, careers, friendships, and family situations change. Be particularly aware of what is happening when you suddenly start developing a brand new Habit or Routine.

One cold winter morning, I had a cup of coffee. I was feeling tired so I had a second cup and then a third. It was lovely. I felt indulgent and warm inside. I went ahead and had three cups the next morning and then the next; before I knew it, I had another Habit/Routine. As soon as I realized what had happened, I decided that I did not want to continue to have three cups of coffee each morning. It was difficult to return to my previous Routine of having one or two cups of coffee in the mornings before work. It is easier to create a Habit that brings with it a sense of comfort or pleasure than to give up a Habit and find another way to meet your needs.

Avoid the Extremes

When you are in the middle of life as a healthy, average size person, it is a good rule of thumb to avoid the extremes. Balance is the key that will keep you calm and feeling a sense of control over what you are eating, what you are doing with your time, and how you are interacting with other people. When you find yourself living in the extreme, such as going out to dinner nightly, taking your children to daily sports activities, working endless amounts of overtime, or volunteering for too many things, you need to stop for a moment and evaluate any new HRRTs you may have developed that could be putting your healthy, average size body at risk.

We all want a perfect ending and a promise that we will never have to think about weight or food issues again. But dear reader, change is inevitable, as we go through the stages of our lives. Managing these changes in MicroSteps provides us with the opportunity to continue to develop healthy HRRTs and to help our children, spouse, family, and friends grow with us. Learning to manage your HRRTs as a way of life is the *lifestyle change* that brings us joy as we continue to live life in the mainstream free of obesity.

CHAPTER 13

Practice Does Not Make Perfect:

The End of Living Large for Children and Teens

RINGING IN MY EARS, I can still hear the clear voice of my high school choir director shouting, "Practice does not make perfect; it makes permanent! Now try that measure again and this time listen to the piano."

This declaration generally came during a rehearsal in which we were making the same mistake repeatedly. He worked us hard but he was also the reason we won so many awards. He had a point. The things you do repeatedly become a Habit, Routine, Ritual, or Tradition and frequently a permanent way of behaving. They become your lifestyle and the lifestyle of your family.

As discussed in earlier chapters, we create Habits out of need, desire, comfort, and perceived necessity. One morning I got up to fix my coffee before work and discovered I was completely out. No problem, I just left the house a little early so that I'd have time to stop and buy a coffee on the way to work. I did this for a week or so until I could make the time to go to the grocery store. Even after I started making my coffee at home again, I felt uneasy as I drove past the coffee shop. It was difficult to drive past and not stop. Their coffee was special and better than mine was. My uneasy feeling and desire to have the special coffee happened because I had created a new Habit or Routine. There is nothing wrong with leaving early and stopping buy my special coffee; this is just an example of how easily we create Habits and Routines.

Some people get into a Habit of simply agreeing when friends suggest pizza for lunch, instead of saying they would prefer to go out for a healthier meal. You may find yourself buying the same shampoo your mother bought and never consider a better brand. It is common to buy the same brands you got used to as a child. To avoid passing unhealthy Habits, Routines, Rituals, or Traditions down to your children, it is necessary to keep an eye on your daily activities and choices. By increasing awareness, you can make sure you are creating healthy HRRTs.

About twenty years ago, I remember working as a Licensed Marriage and Family Therapist with a ten-year-old boy who brought McDonald's French fries to every therapy session. The Routine was that he and his mother would run through the McDonald's right after school for his French fries. I remember it well because the smell made doing therapy a challenge. His session was at 3:30PM right when you are getting hungry for that afternoon pick-me-up. I also remember driving through McDonald's at 9PM to get my own French fries and more after the last session of the evening. Habits and Routines! They are powerful but we do not have to let them control us.

Are your children in the Habit of going to school without eating breakfast? Do your teenagers settle for a soda and chips from the snack machines at school instead of buying lunch? Have you asked yourself what negative Routines have evolved in your daily family life? They are common in many families.

Instead, imagine this scenario: You go to bed at a reasonable hour, get up in time to share a healthy but simple fifteen minute breakfast with your family, where everyone sits down and eats together. The children experience a calm and nurturing moment before going to school; so do you. The children are learning about nurturing themselves, working on manners, improving conversation skills, and feeling loved each morning before school. What effect would this have on their grades, relationships with peers, and your family life? We have the power to choose our Routines. Imagine a Routine that you think is worth developing and work toward that goal in MicroSteps. Get everyone involved and see what you can do as a family team. I know it won't be easy but the payoff will be enormous.

In my own family growing up, we always had our main meal in the evening. When I got older and moved out on my own, I continued this Routine. After I started losing weight, it occurred to me that I did not need to have a large evening meal of meat, potatoes, and vegetables. Often, I wasn't even that hungry and a bowl of soup or a salad was just as satisfying. Nonetheless, when I first started changing this old Routine, I found myself still missing the large evening meal. I would have the soup or salad and then began to crave comfort foods such as chips, desserts, or other such snacks. I was not physically hungry but I was experiencing an emotional hunger created by my deeply imbedded family Routine that was difficult to manage.

The Family Table

There is so much power in the family table that I hardly know where to begin. Children find comfort in Habits, Routines, Rituals, and Traditions perhaps even more than adults do. Habits, Routines, Rituals, and Traditions give children a sense of belonging and safety, the things on which they depend. When they leave home as young adults, their HRRTs accompany them and guide them. The family table is a major part of HRRT development for children, adolescents, and young adults.

I like to think of the family table as a classroom. This is the perfect opportunity for children to learn basic table manners and healthy food choices. How many times have you had to remind your child that the dinner table is not the time for telling disgusting stories or jokes? It is easier to teach these lessons around the table than in front of the television. What are our children learning if they're eating breakfast in the car on the way to school while practicing Spelling Words? They are not learning table manners or giving thought to what they are eating. They are not learning how to enjoy a healthy meal with appropriate family conversation. Success at the family table provides social skills and establishes a sense of confidence, while increasing self-esteem. Remembering that the family table is a classroom, can remind us to teach the lessons our children require to maintain their healthy, average size bodies as well as provide the skills needed to confidently attend any social or career event.

Eating as a family also provides you with an opportunity to be a role model for your children. They observe what you choose to eat and *how* you eat. Are you grabbing junk food as you run out the door? Are you shoving down that fast food instead of eating a healthy meal? Your children are watching, they are copying you, and they will develop their Habits, Routines, Rituals, and Traditions from your example.

One night some years ago, I had dinner with the family of a close friend. I was dismayed as I watched her children reach across the table and use the same forks they were eating with to get seconds from the serving bowls, sometimes even taking a few bites out of the serving bowl first instead of serving themselves and eating off their own plates. One teenager even scooped out some mashed potatoes with his fingers and ate off his fingers! This is a classic example where practice does not make perfect. I looked over at the mother and she said, "It is okay. We're family. They are at home."

The problem with this approach is that what you do at home, you will do outside the home. Allowing this kind of behavior doesn't teach children the manners they need for life. It doesn't teach them to respect boundaries of others or to control their impulses. In the above example, the children took the easy way out by eating out of the serving dish, and in so doing they not only disrespected the others at the table, but they also shared their germs with them.

Years later, I met these children again. By this time, they were in college; but their manners had not improved. They didn't even seem to notice when other people around them stared at them in disbelief over their rude behavior and disregard for basic manners.

It is never too early or too late to begin a family table Routine. If your family has not been used to eating together, then it may take some time to make these changes, but start somewhere. You may not be able to eat every meal together as a family. Unfortunately, family schedules can be a challenge. Begin where you can and build slowly, remembering how well MicroSteps worked for you with your own eating. It makes no sense to say to your teenagers, "You will have to give up the Friday night football game to eat dinner with your family." That will not work and you will have a fight on your hands. Depending on the ages of your children, sit down, talk with your family, and come up with a plan together. Start with only one meal a week if you have to, but start somewhere and build in MicroSteps.

At every meal, our children are learning how to communicate, how to make nutritional choices, social skills, and table manners. Everything, for better or worse, is part of their education. Parents, teachers, peers, and other adults all have a significant influence in this learning. It may take a village but parents are the biggest influence and the ball is in your court.

Birth to Toddler

Your child begins a relationship with food from birth. From day one, an infant learns either to trust that the food will be there or to feel anxious when hungry. They either learn that it is safe to cry and crying brings help, that crying does not bring help, or that it even gets them hurt. This is the time, from birth to preschool, when you as a parent have tremendous power to influence your children's Habits, Routines, Rituals, and Traditions.

If your children have learned from birth to trust that food will be there, they'll feel safe trusting that food will be there when they are hungry. As they get older, chances are good that they won't be overeating out of anxiety or fear. Since you met their needs during infancy, they'll probably never experience that panic, often subconscious, that *"This is my last meal!"* There is no need to overeat at meals because the assumption will be that there are more meals in the future.

Years ago, I met a young boy who was adopted at the age of six by a wonderful family. His first six years had included severe neglect and going without food. His adoptive mother said she was struggling to keep food out of his bedroom. She said he was hiding food in the closets, under the pillows, in the drawers, and in his school backpack. This is an extreme situation but you get the idea. It took a lot of work to help this little boy trust that food would be there for him and he did not need to hide it or hoard for future meals.

Infants learn from birth what to expect from the world. An infant ignored in the crib, crying from hunger, is developing anxiety about how to get needs met. If the person feeding the child is angry, rough, wants the infant to finish quickly, or removes the food before the infant is finished, the infant is learning lessons that will become part of his or her relationship to food.

Every feeding teaches the infant. They learn from how quickly the caregiver responds, from the attitude of the caregiver, from the amount of food provided, and from which foods are provided along the way as they grow older. When we ignore an infant's basic need for food, the baby may eat faster, eat more when food is finally given, or develop anxiety issues about never wanting to be hungry. From birth to toddler years, we have a powerful opportunity to help our little ones develop a healthy relationship with food.

A friend of mine gave birth to adorable twin boys. When they were newly born, I would go to her house to help her with the feedings. I noticed that my friend anticipated their feeding needs and made sure she fed them as soon as they began to act hungry. She did not make them wait while she prepared their bottles or prepared to nurse them. She was ready when they were ready. She always had someone else in the house to assist her so that one of the boys did not have to wait while the other was having a bottle. She pumped so that they had breast milk in bottles and other people could help with the feedings. The babies could count on timely meals. They did not have to cry in frustration while hungry. She continued this consistent meal-time Routine throughout their first year and it has paid off. They are active healthy toddlers and appear to have developed a healthy relationship with food, enjoying the family table.

As babies grow into toddlers, they begin to eat solid foods, and start learning about the world. It is important to expose them to different tastes, textures, and smells. Allowing a toddler to eat finger foods without help, regardless how messy it gets, is a great MicroStep to building interest in taste, texture, fruits, and vegetables. This provides an opportunity to make choices and build confidence.

When you ask, "Do you want a cracker?" If they reach for it, they have made a choice. Yes, it will be messy but messy is okay at this stage. It is a tiny choice and a wee bit of self-feeding; however, it is the first MicroStep to independence in making healthy food choices to support a healthy, average size body.

I remember watching a teenage mother trying to feed her eighteen-month-old son. The child was sitting in a high chair. The mother was talking to her friends in the kitchen, while putting bites of baby food into his mouth. Without noticing that the food was not staying in his mouth, that it was getting all over his clothes, or that he had rubbed it into his eyes, the mother just continued to chat with her friends. When the little fellow began to cry, the mother looked at him and said, "I guess he's not hungry." She roughly cleaned him, gave him a bottle so that he would stop crying, and started to put him to bed. Fortunately, his grandmother was nearby and asked if she could try to feed him.

Grandma had a different approach. She calmed the child, cleaned him up, and put him back in the high chair. She then sat her own chair in front of the baby and smiled as she carefully spooned strained chicken and green beans into his little mouth. She talked to the little one and told him how good the food was. He smiled back. She kept the baby and his high chair clean as she fed him. Grandma made sure the food did not get in his eyes and that each bite was small enough so that it stayed in his mouth. He ate the food without a problem. He learned that eating is pleasant and the chicken and green beans were satisfying. He did not feel ignored or frustrated, and had no need to cry.

The baby was learning about eating without making a mess, about satisfying your tummy with healthy foods, and about appropriate social interaction for his stage of life. Grandma knew that the lessons begin at birth. The young mother was still a teenager with some things to learn. She was watching as Grandma taught her lessons.

Toddlers to Preschool

Do you wait until your car runs out of gas before you refuel? I don't, at least not intentionally. We'd never want to be in the middle of a trip and run out of gas. Then why do people so often wait until they are out of energy and feel hungry, even to the point of starving, before eating?

Often, the idea that food is fuel is not even considered. While we want our children to experience waiting until they are hungry to eat, we do not want them to wait until they are extremely hungry, physically tired, and grabbing candy or chips just to tide them over until dinner. Meeting a toddler's needs in a timely and appropriate manner helps trust grow. This creates young Habits for a healthy relationship with food as they mature.

As you teach your children that food is the fuel we need to help our bodies run, jump, play, and enjoy life, you are helping them develop the Habit of eating to nurture and fuel their body, not to solve emotional problems or reduce stress. Do not give a child food to stop them from crying, unless the child is crying out of hunger. It is important to help children learn how to feel comfort and reduce stress without using food as a drug, in other words, self-medicating. How many times do you hear a parent say, "If you will be good, I will take you to McDonald's?" What is the message? The message is that food is a reward, a fun activity, a social event, and almost anything but fuel to keep the body working properly. By the time a child is three years old, these lessons are well learned Habits.

That's not to say you shouldn't make food an important part of socialization and interpersonal interactions. Naturally, there will be festive times with hot dogs and ice cream at the birthday party. You are just giving them a deeper foundation in their relationship with food so that they are not at the party just for the food. They are merely enjoying the food as they celebrate a friend's birthday and play with peers. How many times, as an adult, did you go to a potluck and all you could think about was what you were eating? I know. I've been there. It's better when you can enjoy the conversations and spending time with other people; the food takes second place, even though you enjoy some of the food as well. When we experience food as fuel, then it is only natural to stop eating when you feel full, leaving you free to enjoy life and relationships.

As babies turn into toddlers and are able to indicate choices about what foods they like and dislike, we have endless opportunities to engage in teachable moments. This is the time to begin to name the foods and give children many new choices about what they want to eat. If you are making frozen vegetables for dinner, you might show your child two packages and ask, "Shall we have carrots or peas tonight?" Then agree with the child and prepare his or her choice. A child is more likely to eat the chosen vegetable and this helps build his confidence and pride in himself. I am not saying give endless choices. By choosing a category such as fruit, vegetables, or meat and then identifying two options in that category, the child has a choice but you are still controlling his basic diet. After all, we are talking about toddlers. The goal is to help the child begin to identify foods and learn to make healthy choices with confidence. As the child ages, food choices become more complex; however, the confidence you are nurturing is building healthy Habits long before the options become unhealthy ones.

Many of us grew up thinking of food as a pleasurable experience and social event; unless, we were poor with parents who struggled to just put food on the table. Today, almost from the beginning, we tell children that the foods they usually want are not good for them and will make them fat or unhealthy. This creates an adversarial relationship with food; deeply imprinted in the HRRTs so that it dictates behavior that can last throughout life. The goal is to help our children *want* to eat the healthy foods, rather than to think of any food as off limits and recognize that some foods are eaten as exceptions to Routine meals. We want children to think of foods as a pleasant way of refueling.

Toddlers need to experience a wide variety of healthy foods so that they develop a taste for healthy choices. They need to see you eating a wide variety of healthy foods as well. They also need to learn how to eat with age-appropriate manners and have age-appropriate social interactions at the dinner table. By seeing you try new things, it will give them the courage to try new foods. As they listen to the adults at the table speaking respectfully to each other, demonstrating love and support, they grow up being able to do the same thing.

As your babies grow into toddlers, notice how they are more able to do some things on their own. At snack time you might offer a choice between two healthy fruits or snacks. Have them say the name of it before they start to eat. This helps them learn how to make healthy choices which will give them confidence. Toddlers who have the beginning skills of identifying foods and making some simple healthy choices are more confident as they venture out into their elementary years. Because they have a Habit of making healthy choices from the early years, doing the same thing will be a no-brainer for them when they get to the school cafeteria.

I was at the birthday party for the two-year-old daughter of a colleague. It took place in the neighborhood park. There was pizza, cakes, and a vegetable tray on the table. The little girl, age two, walked over and took a piece of a pizza. She took a bite, laid it down, then reached over, and grabbed a broccoli. She munched on the broccoli as she played with her friends. Repeatedly, she came back for another of those delicious vegetables and took one after another, preferring the broccoli, as she played around the park. Yes, she still ate a bite of pizza now and then but she clearly enjoyed the vegetables as well. No one was telling her what to eat. She likely had a Habit of eating vegetables. I never saw her eat the cake.

Years ago, a close friend of mine had a three-year-old son who seemed to have a strong reaction to sugar. While his mother was shopping at the local supermarket, the youngster wandered off. He was famous for wandering off. The manager, seeing that the boy appeared to be lost, called for the mother over the loud speaker. While waiting for her to come retrieve the lost child, the manager offered the young boy a candy. The three year old shocked and amused everyone who was nearby when he not only declined the candy, but also explained that it made him too hyperactive and he would be eating dinner soon.

Getting children involved in safe food preparation activities at home, so they learn to make healthy choices and develop a sense of confidence about nutrition is helpful in the development of healthy HRRTs. You might encourage the three year old to bring you the loaf of bread, take it out of the package, and spread the peanut butter on the bread with a child-safe knife. They might be able to take the salad out of the package and put it in the bowls. This is of course after washing hands. A toddler can help put the napkins on the table and make sure everyone in the house knows when dinner is ready. You will find a way, if your goal is to help them build self-esteem, confidence, and develop healthy HRRTs.

My favorite parenting observation occurred when I was in a checkout line at Gelson's Grocery Store in Los Angeles. In the line to my left was a mother with a little boy. He appeared to be about two years old and was sitting in the child's seat part of her cart. As the mother moved closer to the cash register, the child reached for a candy bar that was on a nearby shelf. She told him that he could not have it because they were going to eat lunch soon. He started to cry, kick his feet, and scream loudly about how much he wanted the candy. The mother simply pulled the cart back so he could not reach the candy. She protected the child so he could not hurt himself or her as he kicked and screamed. She waited patiently for two or three minutes until he stopped screaming. When he quieted, she reached her arms around him and said, "That was hard, wasn't it." He leaned into her chest, she hugged him, and they moved to the register to checkout. Not only did her parenting impress me but also her confidence. She did not seem to care that people were staring; she just did her job and did is brilliantly. She taught him that feelings are okay, that you don't eat candy for lunch, and that she was there for him. She was gentle, kind, and clear.

Elementary School

The elementary school years are the perfect time for a child to learn the basic food groups. This helps them identify a healthy meal. These years are a wonderful time to learn because they are like little sponges. They like to learn and will believe what you tell them. So tell them the truth about foods and help them find healthy tasty choices for school lunches and meals at home.

One challenge during these years is that parents are busy. Often, both parents are working; the children have extracurricular activities, play dates, birthday parties of friends, and there are numerous other demands on the family time. It's tempting for parents to resort to driving through the nearest fast food restaurant to grab a quick breakfast on the way to school or dinner on the way home. Worse yet, the parent allows the child to skip breakfast altogether. Skipping breakfast is not a good idea if you want your children to function well mentally and make good grades. Eating healthy non-processed foods makes a big difference for children who are trying to do schoolwork. You know how grouchy children can be when hungry for dinner. The same thing happens when they are hungry at school. They are grouchy, not able to focus, and more likely to misbehave in class. Those drive-through meals are rarely able to provide the nutritional support needed to get a child through a school day.

The challenges are understandable and there is no perfect parent. As a mother or father who has worked hard all day, you are tired. You just want to get the kids fed, homework finished, baths done, and the little darlings in bed for the night so you can finally have a moment of peace for yourself. It is difficult to plan, cook, and teach nutrition, while trying to survive the daily stress of raising your kids and earning a living; however, the consequences of not doing so are severe and could leave your family paying the price for years and years to come.

There is no magic wand to make this time of life easy or simple for the parents; however, there are ways to keep the family eating healthy, while building those all important Habits, Routines, Rituals, and Traditions. If you have begun your own journey of the HRRTs, look for natural ways to include your children and family so that it is not just your journey but also that of your family. You cannot teach your children to make healthy choices if you are not living that way yourself.

Imagine your child coming home from school, asking you for a snack and you say, go do homework, because you are preparing dinner. Your child is tired after a long day at school, grouchy from hunger, doesn't feel up to doing homework, and the evening begins on a negative note. You're tired too and everyone ends up fussing and miserable.

On the other hand, imagine your child coming home hungry, finding a drawer in the kitchen that is just the right height for him, and seeing it loaded with healthy, high protein small snacks, nothing over 100 calories, nothing that will spoil his dinner. He grabs something, enjoys it, and gets on with whatever is next on the agenda, most likely homework. The drawer becomes a Habit that builds energy and always happens just before homework. Since dinner comes after homework, the Routine is clear and expectations for a great family evening are high. You might even enjoy one of those healthy snacks yourself to give you the energy to prepare a nutritious dinner and help with your child's homework at the same time.

Taking the time to buy groceries and plan meals for the week will reduce turning to fast food for survival. Stocking the kitchen with simple, easy to prepare, easy to grab, healthy food not only makes it easier to manage your weight but your children will be developing healthy Habits. The notion of planning and preparing ahead of time is a Habit that will carry over into the life of your children on many levels. How about the project that is due next month? Perhaps, as a family who plans and prepares, your child will develop that lifestyle and you will even see grades improve. You never know. It is not only about food; it is about living a lifestyle that supports a healthy, average size body.

As children get older, it is the perfect time for them to learn to make their own lunches, assist you even more in preparing meals, and develop a sense of confidence about taking care of their own hunger. This will go a long way to keeping them on track with healthy eating as they turn into teenagers. Remember, we are creatures of Habits, Routines, Rituals, and Traditions. Your children will find comfort in the HRRTs you establish and turn to those as they turn into teenagers.

After helping my mother in the kitchen almost from the day I could walk, I cooked my first meal at age nine. The meal consisted of baked Spam that I took out of the can, put on a cake pan, and baked in a 350-degree oven to get it hot and brown. I also made mashed potatoes, green beans, and tomato juice. It was simple, easy to cook, and I was able to do it all by myself.

My mother had been teaching me how to make mashed potatoes for years. I would sit and peal them while she made the rest of the dinner. She taught me how to use the knife safely so that I could peal and slice the potatoes for boiling. I knew just how high to keep the burner after they began to boil so they would not boil over. She showed me how to do this numerous times. She taught me how to test them with a fork to know when they were done. She taught me to pour some salt in my palm and judge just how much to put in the potatoes. I knew how to turn the oven on because she had allowed me to help her do it many times. The Spam dinner was not a fancy meal but I could do it without help and my family said it was good. The green beans came from a can but that is what we used back in those days. I smile now when I think of how important and grown up I felt at the time.

Without knowing it, my mother had been teaching me to cook in MicroSteps. There were simple steps to the meal that she had been teaching me long before I tried to cook a complete dinner. When she was cooking dinner, she would ask me to turn on the oven, open a can, pour the milk, or stir the soup. I had learned how to open the can of Spam, how to use the can opener for the green beans, how to pour juice into a glass without spilling it, how to use a pot holder to prevent getting burned—and to only turn on the oven when she was in the house and had given me permission.

Okay, I confess. My mother was sitting nearby watching and supporting me as I made my first meal. You see, she was pregnant with my little sister and needed to be off her feet. I was happy to help; she was sitting and ironing as I cooked dinner. She tells me that she was watching closely.

My mother was not necessarily teaching me about nutrition or healthy eating to support an average size body; however, she definitely used MicroSteps to teach me how to cook, how to read a recipe, and how to be confident in food preparation. Years later, it would be those cooking skills that helped me discover how to prepare and enjoy healthy foods.

Adolescents

Teenagers are prone to resist everything their parents say, so getting them to eat healthy meals is one of the greatest challenges of parenting. The foundation you have laid down since birth is going to pay off in major ways when your child reaches adolescence. Teenagers who have already developed healthy Habits, Routines, Rituals, and Traditions related to what they eat, where they eat, with whom they eat, and how much they eat, may continue to eat fairly healthy meals, at least when their friends are not looking. While it is never too late to eliminate unhealthy HRRTs or to create healthy ones, it is much easier to develop those healthy HRRTs in the first place.

If your teenager has a Habit of helping you prepare meals, it will be natural to simply increase their skill levels and then one day you will be able to text your teenager, "Hi Sweetie, I'm running late tonight, would you please roast the chicken for dinner?" He or she will have watched you, helped you season it many times, turned the oven on for you in the past, and helped you check the internal temperature to make sure it's ready. It won't be a problem for your teen to do it when you are late getting home since the Routine of helping you prepare meals is already in place, deeply embedded in memories from childhood. Later, they can do it for themselves in their own home. Now, that is a HRRT to be treasured. Imagine all these healthy HRRTs passed down generation to generation.

Suppose that you are just starting to catch onto the power of the HRRTs and your teenager is not interested in joining the team. You cannot go back to his or her infancy or childhood and build a foundation. While you may feel there's no hope, don't give up. Do you remember those MicroSteps from earlier chapters? This is your chance to slip in a MicroStep to help build some of those healthy eating Habits. Decide what Habit or Routine you want to establish. Break it into MicroSteps. Pick the easiest and start there. Make it so easy that there is no chance for failure.

A good example of this might be adding a twist to pizza night. Suppose, just for fun, that your teenage son likes to have pizza on Friday nights before he and his friends go to the football game at their high school. His two best friends always come over and they eat together. In the past, they have been eating the unhealthy greasy pies he orders from the local pizza restaurant. One night, before he can resist, take out a variety of delicious looking ingredients you've already prepared ahead of time. Suggest that he make a "homemade pizza" and ask him what he wants on it. You can start him out with a crust you've also made ahead of time so there is no chance of failure. You encourage him and his friends to make their pizzas their own way and give them plenty of healthy ingredients. They are suddenly in charge, *the teen dream.*

Point out to your teen this is all going to take him less time than ordering out and the homemade one will be larger and better. They can eat twice as much! Teenage boys love this. You simply give them Olive Oil instead of unhealthy oils, healthy tomato sauce, some favorite cheeses, a variety of vegetables, and their favorite lean meats for toppings. Surprisingly you have a fresh salad already made in the refrigerator. You offer it. This may not be the world's healthiest meal but it is far better than that fast food he and his friends have been eating. It is free of preservatives, the ingredients that we cannot pronounce, and trans fats. It is a MicroStep.

The idea here is that you are choosing foods he already likes but making them healthier. You respected his independent spirit by letting him make the pizza himself but choosing something fail-proof so that he feels successful in front of his friends. You will leave them alone with simple directions but check in from time to time. Tell them how great they are doing and do not look at the messy kitchen. Save cleanup duty for another MicroStep.

It is a beginning. The beginning MicroStep means that at least one night a week your teen is not eating fast food and has a couple servings of vegetables on the pizza, perhaps even some salad. It's a start. Once this has become the new Tradition for Friday nights before the game, think of another MicroStep that will help create healthy eating. Slip the MicroSteps in a little bit at a time. Do not worry, although it may take a while to have your teen eating healthy. Making changes in MicroSteps will help prevent the resistance, anxiety, and anger often seen in teenagers. You cannot eliminate unhealthy HRRTs overnight.

Eventually, your teen might learn to go to the store, buy the ingredients, prep the toppings, make the pizza, and clean up after they are finished eating. There are many MicroSteps involved so take your time and let them evolve slowly. This is only one example. I am sure you can think of many ways to engage your teens in developing HRRTs for healthier eating.

From the day I got my driver's license, my mother allowed me to do a lot of the grocery shopping. She would give me a list and send me on my way. She could do that because I had spent years going to the grocery store with her, learning which brands she liked, and how to choose the best produce. Again, I was not learning about nutrition at that time because we were living in Texas and eating my mother's delicious Southern style cooking. To this day, I can fry chicken with the best of them and make cream gravy with the drippings from the chicken. I do not do it often but I use the skills I learned to make many healthy foods.

My mother could not teach what she, at that time, did not know; however, she did teach me how to cook and I am grateful. I have been able to use the skills that I learned in her kitchen to help me create my own HRRTS for healthy eating. You can begin to teach your children skills for healthy eating at any age. All you need to do is start.

College and Young Adult Years

By the time your kids are in college, you may think it's too late to make changes, but believe me you still have influence. After all, they do come home for visits and holidays. You are still an example for them. Never give up; just keep trying in Micro-Steps. Have a conversation about your own progress; tell them what you are learning. Young adults and college students who were lucky enough to have healthy HRRTs passed down to them since they were infants are best prepared to live a healthy adult life. They are more likely to pass those skills down to their own children; however, it is never too late. You developed healthy HRRTs as an adult and so can they.

A friend of mine has a son who is now in his early twenties. He spent his childhood refusing to eat anything but hotdogs, plain sandwich meats, green beans out of a can, string cheese, raw carrots, and pepperoni pizza. He left home to go to college and had meals in the school cafeteria the first year, while living in the dormitory. He then resorted to eating at a Subway sandwich shop a couple of times a day for the next couple of years, while living in an apartment with friends. He had no cooking skills and didn't know how to shop for food. He resorted to fast food most of the time, even though he lived in his own apartment with a kitchen available. This was expensive and unhealthy. He loved it when he had a home cooked meal at family events. These did not happen often enough for him.

He is a perfect example of a young adult who was not prepared to meet his own nutritional needs. While still in college, this young man and his girlfriend became pregnant. Although the couple broke up, they both took care of their adorable young son. The young man became concerned about the gap in his food knowledge. He took responsibility for learning about nutrition, food preparation, and became a fine father. The last time I spoke with him, he had mastered spaghetti and meatballs for his son. Now, I call that progress!

Breaking the Cycle of Obesity One Family at a Time

At the age of fifty-nine, I tasted my first mango! It was delicious. Imagine the number of years I spent not knowing the taste of a mango. It was simple. My family did not eat mangos. We ate apples, oranges, bananas, grapes, and peaches. My parents did not give me mango when I was a child and thus I did not have an interest in it until recently. A Food Network show on television stimulated my interest and I bought one. I knew how to cut it because of that show. I ate it and loved it. I may have had mango in foods over the years but did not know that it was in the ingredients. It is so nutritious, delicious, low in calories, and was right there all the time, waiting to help me maintain a healthy, average size body. My point is that children will not know all the wonderful choices that are out there if you do not expose them to a wide variety of foods.

While this chapter focuses on creating healthy eating HRRTs, it is important to help your children develop healthy lifestyles in terms of getting up, getting out, and moving. Productive Exercise is also important for children and teenagers.

Families that are active from the time the child is born are more likely to produce adults that are active and enjoy a wide variety of physical and social activities. The world will have one less couch potato or computer game addict!

Start by taking your infant for a walk in the stroller. This will get you moving and the baby will be learning that taking a walk is a fun Habit. We want our children to develop healthy eating HRRTs but it can't stop there. They need healthy HRRTs in all areas of their lives. This includes social, emotional, intellectual, and physical.

I copied the following Tweet from Clinton Kelly, costar of *What Not to Wear* and *The Chew;* "Babysitting my awesome nephews tonight—and already looking forward to our dinner of pizza, mac & cheese and ice cream!" Now, while there is nothing wrong with this as an occasional menu, hopefully he was preparing healthier versions of these timeless kid foods.

My thought is that instead of identifying certain foods as kid foods, we need to bring the children into the world of variety where there are wonderful healthy foods that are not loaded with preservatives and trans fats, but include lean meats with lots of fresh vegetables and fruits. Start when they are young and they will develop healthy cravings for a wide variety of whole well made foods.

If MicroSteps work for adults who have deeply embedded HRRTs, they will work for children of all ages; their young HRRTs are open to creation. The younger the child when you start the better—but it is never too late. Go for it! It is time to create a healthy generation.

Chapter 14

A New Way of Living

AT THE AGE OF SIXTY-THREE, I am at last comfortable in my own skin. I am no longer living large but absolutely living better and enjoying a new lifestyle. If you recall, it was at age fifty that I gave up dieting and decided to accept being obese. As of today, I have lost eighty pounds from my greatest weight of 315. The medical community still labels me as obese. It doesn't matter because I feel like an average size person. I also feel healthier now that I am smaller. Of course, I am still taking MicroSteps to lose an additional fifty to sixty pounds—my personal target weight. To be completely honest with you, I have come to enjoy taking MicroSteps to help me achieve improved health and weight loss. I don't care how long it takes to get to my target weight. I am on the downside of the mountain and enjoying the slope.

At this point, I just want to be absorbed into the mainstream of life and to feel normal. I don't need people to celebrate my weight loss. I don't particularly enjoy it when people look at me with the "I can't believe it! You've lost so much weight! How did you do it? WOW!" My heart sings when my weight goes unnoticed.

At 315 pounds, I could not hide my obesity. My secret issues with food were as *out there* as a YouTube gone viral. Today I am at peace knowing that my obesity and food issues are resolved and no longer announcing my shame. When people simply assume that I'm just another healthy person of average size, I rejoice inside my heart. I am *average*. The obesity is past. I am done with that. I am okay with my current weight, relieved that the obesity is gone, and have a strong sense of persistence driving me to my target weight as I continue living in the land of MicroSteps.

Do not let yourself get cocky at this stage of the journey! It is far too easy to create new unhealthy HRRTs or return to old ones. For instance, I stopped eating those jars of Hormel Real Bacon Bits a long time ago. They are not a good source of nutrition and seem like empty calories. I suspect they are unhealthy as well. This past Christmas, I was making a recipe that called for bacon crumbled on the top. I was in a hurry and grabbed a jar of the Hormel Real Bacon Bits off the shelf instead, telling myself that at least I would not have to smell the bacon cooking or start craving bacon.

That was all it took for me to start sprinkling bacon bits on top of my eggs each morning, crave a mayonnaise, tomato, and bacon bit sandwich, and then add bacon bits to my next grocery list. As discussed in previous chapters, whatever you do on a daily basis is likely to become a Habit, Routine, Ritual, or Tradition. Now, I am not saying that you should stop eating bacon or bacon bits. Eat whatever you want but be aware that you are creating Habits, Routines, Rituals, and Traditions.

Those bacon bits could have derailed me, had I not become aware. Instead, I decided that it would be okay to finish the jar. I did not buy another jar at that time but I might buy one again someday. It's not about bacon bits; it is about my daily Habits and Routines. I finished the jar slowly by having them on my eggs only every other day— varying my breakfast Routine. That seemed to keep in check my desire to buy more jars so that I could sprinkle them on my eggs every morning. Varying my breakfast Routine helped me remember that I like my eggs without bacon bits as well. You are not powerless to your Habits, Routines, Rituals or Traditions, as long as you remember that you can change them in MicroSteps, find a way to remain encouraged, and use the tools you have learned along the way.

Average Size

While I have given away most of the clothes that are from my days of being 315 pounds, every now and then I go into my closet and take a quick look at the few left hanging; this helps me remember how valuable my Habits, Routines, Rituals, and Traditions are for keeping my body a healthy, average size. I feel sad when I see a large person struggling to fit into a seat, out of breath from walking, or looking embarrassed by his or her appearance. I remember and know that, but for MicroSteps and changing my unhealthy HRRTs, I would still be that person. Obesity hurts on so many levels. I never want to go back there again.

Often I am in contact with people who have had one of the various weight loss surgeries. I listen to their stories of struggles and say a whisper prayer of thanks that I did not take that road.

Since I am not a medical doctor, I do not want to discuss the risks; however, I encourage anyone who is considering such a treatment for obesity to talk to their doctor and do plenty of their own research. There are people for whom bariatric surgery may be lifesaving; other people say they regret the procedure. A family friend had the surgery, lost over a hundred pounds, and regained all of the weight. She also has problems with vitamin deficiency, since having the procedure.

I meet people struggling with the first one diet plan and then another. They lose weight and then regain it. The unhealthy eating and extreme weight variations damage both their self-esteem and body. Taking MicroSteps to change my unhealthy HRRTs, rescued me, freed me, and gave me back my life. With a bit of sadness for all those years of pain, I remember and I am thankful.

As we conclude this part of our journey together, I want to give you something that I hope will help should you find yourself discouraged. Below is what I say to myself, when I need encouragement in my continued walk— taking MicroSteps to change unhealthy HRRTs.

Supportive Self-Talk

1. If you are not succeeding, make the MicroStep smaller, or even smaller, until you do succeed.

2. Habits, Routines, Rituals, and Traditions are powerful. Keep an eye on them.

3. Portion size matters, even when you are eating a healthy diet. You CAN eat too much healthy food.

4. Are you regretting what you ate yesterday? Let it go. Start with a healthy breakfast and you're back on track.

5. Perfection is not required. You only fail if you quit.

6. You may never be a person who exercises in a GYM but every physical move counts. Wiggle a little and be proud of yourself.

7. Don't give up! If you had one bite of healthy food today, celebrate your success.

8. Celebrate the small stuff! Rejoice in your heart and know you will make it.

9. It does not matter how small the MicroStep is— progress is progress.

10. You are worth it. You can do this. Just don't give up. It will be okay.

If you feel stuck and cannot seem to take those MicroSteps, look at the balance in your overall life. Does something need to change to free you to move forward? MicroSteps will work in any area of your life. It is not just about food. It is about changing your lifestyle forever. It is about living life as a healthy, average size person and not feeling bad about you ever again.

As long as you are managing your Habits, Routines, Rituals, and Traditions, you will eventually get to your healthy, average size body in the mainstream of life. Walk slowly. Enjoy each MicroStep of success. My best to you.

Before and After Headshots

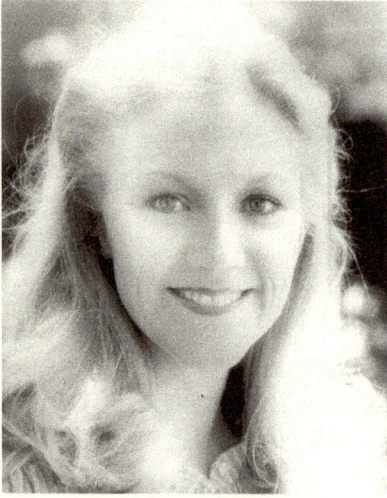

1979, Age 28, 135 lbs.

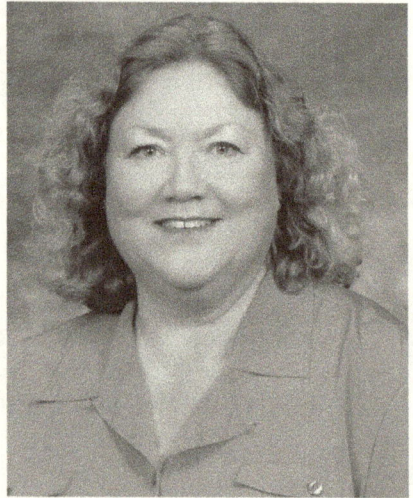

January 2008, Age 57, 315 lbs.

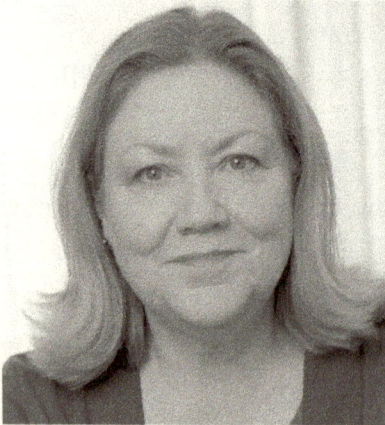

November 2014, Age 63, 234 lbs.
"I'm back!"

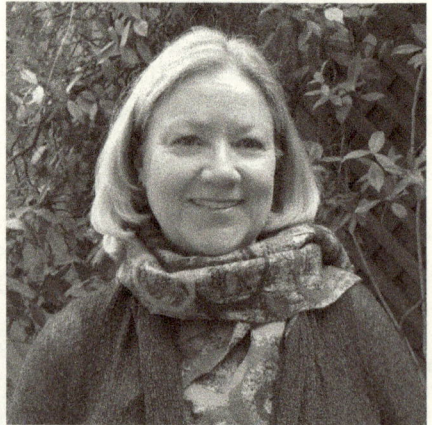

December 2014, Age 63, 234 lbs.
"Feeling good!"

Before and After Full Shots

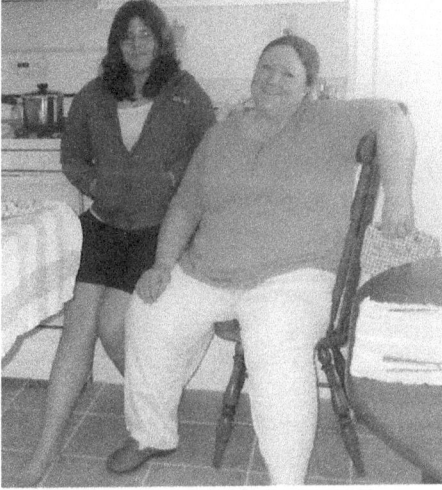

With my niece, Lauren. 2004 or 2005, 315 lbs.
Tired. Low energy.

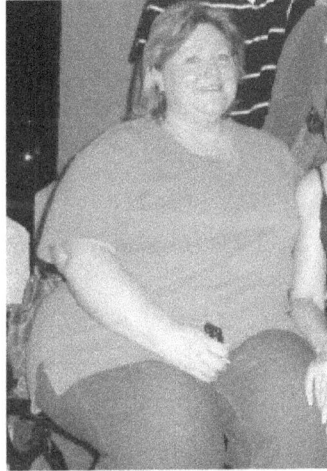

2006, 315 lbs. Miserable.

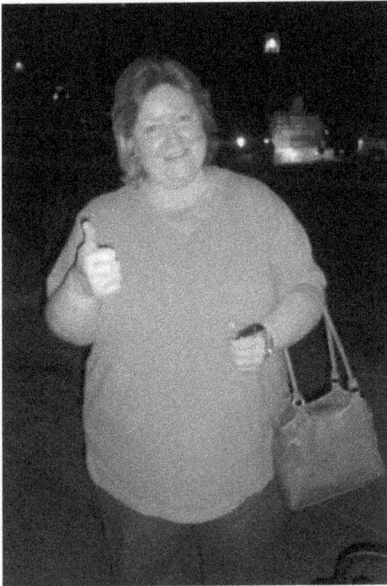

2006, 315 lbs. Humiliated!

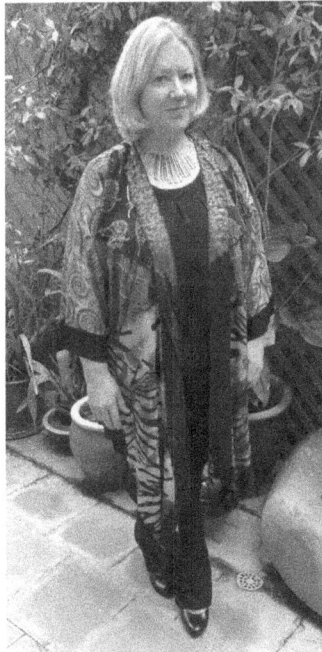

December 2014, Age 63. 234 lbs.
Not at goal weight but back in the
mainstream and loving it!

Recipes and Meal Ideas

Recipes and Meal Ideas

A couple of years ago, with the help of my gardener, I planted my own herb garden. In the past, I would buy fresh herbs and use some, but the rest would spoil before I needed them. Having my own herb garden helps me use fresh herbs as a Routine. As the seasons change so does my little herb garden, bringing me lovely, free, healthy organic herbs. The herbs are right next to a Meyer lemon tree. The lemons and herbs are wonderful to cook with and provide a beautiful view outside the back window.

Having never planted a garden before, I was so excited the first time I made chicken with rosemary and thyme using my own herbs. It was so flavorful! I could not believe that I made it with fresh herbs from my own garden. I had walked outside into my back yard, snipped herbs from the plant, and walked back into the kitchen. I washed them, dried them, and cooked with them. It was easier than going to the grocery store. Why would I ever want fast food again with such wonderful choices!

This simple activity of planting an herb garden helped me in my journey toward a healthy, average size body. I have learned to love taking control of what goes into my body and enjoying the process of creating healthy delicious meals. You do not need to plant an herb garden to make this happen. Remember, it is your journey and you must do what is comfortable for your life situation.

The recipes in this chapter are not diet. I believe they are healthy. They are things I enjoy cooking and eating. My intention is to give you a few ideas and to provide you with a starting point for creating your own healthy meals and eventually healthy HRRTs.

Energy Building Breakfast

As I have said before, I always eat breakfast. Of the various foods I enjoy for breakfast, these three simple meals are my *go to* breakfasts for those days when I am working, in a hurry, or simply not in the mood to cook. They have enough complex carbs and protein to keep me satisfied for at least four hours.

Hard-boiled Egg and Whole Grain Toast with Peanut Butter

- *1-2 eggs*
- *1 slice of whole grain bread*
- *1-2 tablespoons peanut butter (almond butter is also good)*
- *salt*
- *pepper*
- *honey or maple syrup (optional)*

Put the eggs in small saucepan. Add hot water to cover. Turn on the burner. Set a timer for 13 minutes. The time may be different depending on the size of your pan and if you want your eggs hard or soft boiled. When the timer goes off, remove the pan from the burner. Empty out the hot water, place saucepan with eggs under the faucet running cold water and add a few ice cubes. Let them sit about five minutes. Peel them, cut them in half lengthwise, and sprinkle with a little salt and pepper. (You may have your own way of boiling eggs.)

Take one or two slices of whole grain bread. Toast it to your liking. Add peanut butter and enjoy. Some days I even drizzle a bit of honey or maple syrup on the top.

You could substitute almond butter and have a completely different treat for your taste buds. I like to add a few slices of orange or some strawberries to the plate for a little extra nutrition. The bright colors make the plate look like those served in a restaurant. Making it pretty helps me feel nurtured.

When you're buying peanut or almond butter, be sure to read the ingredients. The majority of peanut butter and almond butter brands have trans fats or other oils added. I buy brands that have a little salt and either peanuts or almonds as the only ingredients. They are the brands that you have to stir and keep refrigerated. Once you stir them, if you don't keep them in the refrigerator, they separate again. It is a little more work but so much healthier.

෧෪ ෧෪ ෧෪

Greek Yogurt with Granola

- *½ to 1 cup plain nonfat Greek yogurt*
- *¼ cup granola (keep it healthy, not the kind with candy in it)*
- *¼ cup fresh or frozen blueberries or other fruit*

Take ½ to 1 cup of yogurt. Add a bit of honey to your taste. Stir. Instead of plain, you could use the vanilla flavor and leave out the honey. Put ¼ cup of granola on top. Add blueberries or other fruit on top. Yum!

Oatmeal with Fruit, Nuts, and Maple Syrup

- *steel cut or regular oatmeal*
- *maple syrup*
- *sliced fresh fruit or frozen blueberries*
- *walnuts*
- *butter (optional)*

Make steel cut oatmeal or regular oatmeal (not the instant kind, and not the kind in small packages) according to the directions on the box. I generally have a large bowl because it is so healthy. I like to add some maple syrup, sliced fruits (different fruits depending on the season), and a few chopped walnuts. Frozen blueberries are a favorite and they are always in my freezer. I may even add a tablespoon of real butter. You get to decide how much syrup, fruit, and nuts.

ℰ℘ ℰ℘ ℰ℘

Satisfying Lunch in a Box

Since I generally take my lunch to work, I need some *go to* lunch ideas that are easy to make and easy to eat. Getting out the door on time for work is a challenge so my lunch must be extremely simple to make. When I am working, I think of lunch as fuel and not necessarily the *meal magnificent*. Occasionally, I go out for lunch but listed below are my primary *go to* lunch items.

Fruit Salad

- *fresh fruit*
- *½ lime*

Choose some fruits. Cut them up and put them in a plastic container. Apples, oranges, peaches, pears, tangerines, mango, strawberries, or other berries are all good. Cut the lime in half and squeeze some of the juice on the fruit. Stir and pack in the container. Fruit salad goes really well with a piece of grilled chicken or a sandwich.

You could also grab your favorite nonfat Greek yogurt and toss it into your lunch pail. Be sure to have some blue ice packs in the pail. Into a baggie, add a handful of healthy granola. When it is time to eat, mix it all together. Delicious!

એફ્રે એફ્રે એફ્રે

Simple Sandwich with Vegetables and Fruit

- *2 slices whole grain bread (multigrain is good—the healthiest you can find)*
- *1 slice of cheese (your favorite)*
- *a piece of grilled chicken breast or pork chop*
- *1 tablespoon mustard (or other dressing)*
- *6 or 7 mini carrots or other raw vegetables*
- *1 piece of fruit*

Put the bread and cheese together and stick it into a baggie. Buying pre-sliced cheese will help with portion control. Slice a piece of leftover grilled chicken breast or pork chop and put it in a small plastic baggie. I keep the meat in a baggie and add it to the sandwich just before I eat. Put a little mustard or other dressing in a small container. That way your bread does not get soggy. Throw a few mini carrots, some slices of red bell pepper, an apple or other fruit into baggies and you have lunch.

I like to buy those small condiment containers that the fast food restaurants are so famous for using when they give you meals to go. I buy them at places like Smart & Final. They are inexpensive and make my lunches feel as though I have gone out to eat. I keep them in stock so that I'm always prepared. It helps me feel nurtured and satisfied.

એફે એફે એફે

I got the next idea from my father. He loved ground beef cooked, browned, and mixed into a good ole' southern style milk gravy with salt and black pepper. He called it "SOS." He said they served it in the Army—maybe some of you veterans remember. I shan't tell you what the acronym stood for, since this is a G-Rated book. When I was a child, my mother made it and we enjoyed it over toasted white bread, biscuits, or mashed potatoes. It was amazing but not so healthy. You will see on the following page that I've made a few adjustments. This simple dish brings back lovely memories of family Habits, Routines, Rituals, and Traditions from my southern childhood.

Ground Turkey & Gravy

- 2½ pounds ground turkey (I prefer breast meat)
- 1½ teaspoons poultry seasoning
- 1½ teaspoons salt
- ½ teaspoon black pepper
- 4-5 tablespoons of whole wheat flour (the less flour the thinner the gravy, your preference)
- 2-3 tablespoons canola oil
- 32 oz. Swanson's Chicken Broth, fat free, low sodium

In a small bowl, blend the poultry seasoning with the salt and pepper. Set aside. In a large skillet, add 2 tablespoons canola oil. Turn heat on medium. Crumble in the ground turkey. As you stir the turkey, break it into small pieces. Once completely cooked, remove the turkey from the skillet to a bowl and set aside.

Reduce heat to low or keep on medium, depending on your skillet and stove. Into the skillet, add remaining canola oil and about half of the chicken broth. Whisk the poultry seasoning with the salt and pepper into the broth. Use the whisk to help remove any turkey particles or drippings from the skillet and blend those into the broth as well. Slowly add the remaining broth and flour, whisking together until blended. Hint: A small metal whisk works best. Once the flour and broth are blended, add back into the skillet the cooked turkey.

Cook uncovered on low to medium heat for 5-10 minutes allowing the gravy to thicken. Stir frequently, making sure it does not stick to bottom of pan. Taste and add salt or pepper, if needed. This freezes nicely. It is delicious over brown rice, multigrain toast, egg noodles, whole wheat pasta, or potatoes.

This is not a fancy meal and I doubt that it would impress a Food Network chef but I love it I confess. This is my favorite *take-to-work* lunch. I make it on the weekend, freeze it in individual containers, and take one to work with brown rice that I have frozen in ½ cup containers. I microwave them at work, mix them together, and find they are as tasty and comforting as macaroni and cheese. My little lunch secret is now yours for the taking. I add a few raw vegetables and a piece of fruit to my lunch bag and I am on the road to a healthy, average size body.

۞ ۞ ۞

Ten Lunch Items that Require Very Little Preparation

1. String cheese, individually wrapped

2. Greek Yogurt, any flavor (I eat the yogurt slightly stirred and leave most of the sugary fruit uneaten on the bottom. I also buy the low or nonfat.)

3. Granola bars (Make sure they have healthy ingredients, limit sugar, and no trans fats.)

4. Hardboiled egg, or maybe two (If I take two, I eat only one of the yolks.)

5. Kashi cereal, snack bars, or crackers (Read the ingredients to make sure the ones you choose are not too high in sugar.)

6. Fruit either fresh or frozen (If frozen is your choice, make sure it does not have sugar.)

7. Raw vegetables (Cut and prepare the night before.)

8. A bag of lettuce (Add your raw vegetables and a little container of dressing. You have a salad.)

9. A piece of grilled chicken (I keep these prepared, wrapped individually, and in my freezer. It will likely defrost by noon or you can Microwave it for a few seconds and throw it on bread or a salad.)

10. Soup or chili (Pull out an individual serving container of frozen soup or chili that you have made and saved in your freezer. Microwave for lunch at work.)

You could have some of the above items as a snack around 3:30 in the afternoon if you are hungry and your energy is low. I frequently eat part of my lunch at noon and the rest around 3:30. I also keep some Kashi Bars and a small bag of plain almonds in my office for emergency hunger. I do not want to feel so desperately hungry that I end up at the snack machines in the lounge. In addition, I don't want to be starving when I get home from work. When I am starving, my choices are more impulsive and I tend to snack and then eat a full meal anyway. I prefer prevention. It works for me. You need to develop your own well thought out Routine.

❧ ❧ ❧

Comforting Entrées

While I have a substantial breakfast and satisfying lunch, I am generally hungry for dinner. Some days I want a full meal and other days I just need something light but with a dash of comfort. Below are the recipes of some of my favorite entrées. Of course, they work just as well for a Sunday lunch or anytime you want a substantial meal. By the way, I did not include fish because I am not very good at making fish. When I want fish, I eat out. I'm a psychotherapist—not a chef.

You might want to add sides such as a small salad, delicious steamed vegetables, brown rice, or a small baked potato. If you do not already have one, a rice cooker is a great addition to any kitchen; rice freezes perfectly in small individual size containers. Brown rice or wild rice is a wonderful side dish to many entrees.

Rosemary Thyme Grilled Chicken Breasts

- *6 boneless skinless chicken breasts (large half breast)*
- *¼ cup fresh rosemary finely chopped (about 3 tablespoons dried/crushed)*
- *2 tablespoons fresh thyme finely chopped (about 1½ tablespoons dried)*
- *1 tablespoon garlic powder*
- *1 tablespoon lemon pepper*
- *1-2 teaspoons kosher salt*
- *5-6 tablespoons canola oil*

Into a bowl, add rosemary, thyme, garlic powder, lemon pepper, kosher salt to taste. You do not need a lot of salt because the herbs have a lot of flavor. Just remember three parts rosemary to one part thyme. Whisk the dry ingredients together making a dry rub. You could double the amount of seasonings if it seems there is not enough to cover the chicken. Dry the chicken breasts with a paper towel. Sprinkle the dry rub on each side. In a stainless steel skillet or stovetop grill, put enough canola oil to cover the bottom of pan. Heat the pan and add chicken. On the top of the chicken, drizzle a little canola oil. Cook on medium heat, six to seven minutes each side. Let rest a few minutes and enjoy.

To freeze chicken: Wrap each leftover chicken breast individually in plastic wrap, removing as much air as possible, and place each in a sandwich-size freezer bag. In a gallon-size freezer bag, put as many of the individual bags of chicken as it will hold. Place in freezer for later use. These are great for taking in your lunch to make you feel like you've been nurtured at noon.

⚜ ⚜ ⚜

Pork Chops in Gravy

- *6-8 boneless pork loin chops (may substitute boneless skinless chicken breasts)*
- *4 tablespoons whole wheat flour*
- *salt, lemon pepper, garlic powder to taste*
- *32 oz. Swanson's chicken broth (low sodium, fat free)*
- *2 tablespoon apple cider vinegar*
- *2 tablespoons canola oil*

Sprinkle both sides of the pork chops with Kosher Salt, Garlic Powder, and lemon pepper. In a large skillet, add canola oil. Using medium to high heat, brown both sides of the pork chops. Remove the pork chops from skillet and sit aside.

Adjust heat as needed. In the same skillet add a little of the chicken broth. Whisk the drippings from the pan into the broth. Slowly add the flour and remaining chicken broth; continue whisking while bringing to a boil. Add the apple cider vinegar, a pinch of salt, a sprinkle of garlic powder, and a dash of lemon pepper. Wisk to blend, making a gravy. Add the pork chops into the gravy. Reduce low heat; cook covered for 15 minutes. Stir a couple times to make sure nothing sticks to the bottom of the pan. Taste gravy and add salt or lemon pepper as needed. Cook 5 minutes more. Serve over brown rice, egg noodles, or potatoes.

Freeze leftovers in individual servings by simply putting a pork chop in a plastic container and covering with gravy. It reheats perfectly.

⚜ ⚜ ⚜

Tortilla Chicken Soup

- *6 skinless boned chicken breasts, lightly salted on both sides*
- *1 cup yellow onion diced large*
- *3 tablespoons cilantro dried (if using fresh chop about ¼ cup)*
- *3–4 cloves fresh garlic, minced finely and smashed (or 1½ teaspoons garlic powder)*
- *1–3 tablespoons canola oil*
- *2 teaspoons kosher salt to taste (salt each layer lightly)*
- *2 (32 ounce) containers Swanson chicken broth (low sodium, fat free)*
- *3 (14.5 ounce) cans diced petite tomatoes*
- *½ cup carrots, dice small*
- *1 cup yellow squash diced*
- *2 (7 ounce) cans La Victoria Diced Green Chilies, mild, fire roasted, drained (or 4–5 fresh jalapenos diced small, seeds and veins removed)*
- *¼ teaspoon cumin*
- *3/4 teaspoon chili powder*
- *⅓ cup lime juice*
- *1 (15 ounce) can pinto beans drained and rinsed*
- *2 cups frozen corn*

Grill chicken (stovetop grill, or skillet) in canola oil 5 minutes per side. Allow to cool for about 20 minutes then dice into bite sizes. It will finish cooking later. In the large soup pot, sauté diced onions in canola oil for 2–3 minutes. Add a teaspoon of salt. Add the dried cilantro and mix well with the onions. If using fresh cilantro, wait and add later. Add the minced smashed garlic to the pot. Cook the garlic only until you can smell it, 1-2 minutes. If using garlic powder, add now for 10 seconds only.

Add chicken broth, diced tomatoes, diced chicken, carrots, squash, green chilies, cumin, chili powder, lime juice, black beans, and corn to the pot. Stir gently. Add remainder of kosher salt. If using fresh cilantro, add now. Cover with lid, bring to simmer, cook on lowest possible heat for 20-30 minutes. Let it sit for 10 minutes before serving. Serve in a bowl with a few broken tortilla chips sprinkled on top and other toppings as desired. Freeze leftovers for use later.

Optional Toppings:
- *Tortilla chips (break a few and sprinkle on top of each serving)*
- **Sour cream (just a tablespoon on top of each serving)*
- *Diced fresh avocado (drop in a few in each bowl as you serve)*
- *Shredded Mozzarella cheese (just a little sprinkled on top)*

*Did you know that you could substitute nonfat plain Greek yogurt in place of sour cream? Just stir in a little salt to the plain Greek yogurt and serve as you would sour cream.

Amazing! I generally eat this soup without any toppings. It feels like a comfort food to me.

❧ ❧ ❧

Lemon Pepper Garlic Chicken Breasts

- *6 boneless skinless chicken breasts (may substitute boneless pork loin chops)*
- *garlic powder to taste*
- *lemon pepper to taste*
- *salt to taste*
- *3-4 tablespoons canola oil*

Lay the chicken breasts on paper towels. Dry thoroughly with paper towels. Sprinkle with garlic powder, salt, and lemon pepper on both sides. To a regular size skillet (do not use nonstick) add just enough canola oil to cover the bottom of pan. Heat the skillet. Add chicken. Drizzle a bit of canola oil on the top of each piece of chicken. Cook on each side, medium heat, six to seven minutes or until juices run clear when pierced with a knife. It also works nicely on stovetop grill pan. Let rest a few minutes and enjoy.

By the way, this recipe works equally well with pork chops. Just switch out the chicken for pork chops and everything else stays the same. Once you learn to cook, it becomes easy to take a recipe and switch things up to make it your own. Chicken and pork chops freeze easily, as described earlier with the *Rosemary Thyme Grilled Chicken Breasts*.

Roasted Chicken Legs

- *chicken legs*
- *salt*
- *lemon pepper*
- *garlic powder*
- *canola oil*

Ingredient amounts are to taste and depend on how many chicken legs you cook. I generally cook at least twelve at a time. Sometimes I make a lot more and freeze most of them.

Preheat oven to 375º. Clean the chicken legs and dry with paper towels. Place chicken legs on paper towels. To the dry chicken legs sprinkle salt, lemon pepper, and garlic powder. Do all sides. Go lightly with salt and garlic powder and a little more generous with the lemon pepper. Do not overdo.

Using a glass Pyrex 9" x 13" baking dish, coat the bottom and sides with canola oil. Add the chicken legs to the baking dish. Bake in 375-degree oven uncovered for around one hour or until crispy and juices run clear. It would be 165-170 degrees internal with thermometer. They should start to look brown. Let sit for 10-15 minutes before serving

This type of roasting would also work with any other pieces of chicken or a whole chicken cut into pieces. I would keep the skin on while cooking. I like to cook with the skin on and then eat only a few bites of the skin when eating the chicken. The skin seems to keep it moist.

Freezing Instructions for roasted chicken: Put two or three legs (or one breast) at a time in a sandwich-size freezer bag, trying to remove most of the air. (I don't wrap these in the plastic wrap first because the skin keeps them moist.) Next, take the individual serving bags of chicken, place as many as possible in a gallon-size freezer bag, and place in the freezer. When you are ready to eat them, just take out one of the individual serving bags. You can reheat them in the microwave on medium power for 3-5 minutes or put in the refrigerator to thaw out the night before. Be sure to take them out of the freezer bags before reheating in the microwave. They reheat nicely on a paper plate with a second paper plate covering.

❧ ❧ ❧

Black-Eyed Pea Soup

- *1 pound package of dried black-eyed peas*
- *6-8 cups chicken stock, low sodium & fat free*
- *⅓ cup yellow onion, diced small*
- *2 teaspoons fresh garlic minced (or 1 1/2 teaspoons garlic powder)*
- *1 tablespoon canola oil*
- *1½ teaspoon kosher salt*
- *¼ teaspoon black pepper (or to taste)*
- *Optional: red pepper flakes or a few dashes of hot sauce (not my preference)*

Look carefully at the dried peas, a small handful at a time. Discard any bad peas or small rocks. Set aside. Into the soup pot, drizzle canola oil. Add onions and a dash of salt. Sauté the onions on low heat until they onions turn clear. Add fresh minced garlic. Cook for a few seconds, just until you smell the garlic. If using garlic powder, wait and add with salt. Add 6-8 cups chicken broth, pepper, and salt. Use more broth for more soup-like when done.

Rinse the peas in cool water to remove dust. Do this carefully so as not to damage. Drain and add to the pot. Cover and bring to a boil; immediately, reduce to lowest possible heat. Tilt lid slightly if needed to avoid boiling over. Low simmer about 45–50 minutes or until peas are done but not too soft. Monitor closely so as not to overcook. Time varies with the size of your pan. Taste; adjust salt and pepper, if needed. Serve mixed with wild or brown rice, over a baked potato, or simply by itself with a chunk of cornbread. This is also a great side dish with a sandwich or salad.

꙰ ꙰ ꙰

I cook these and other comforting foods as a Routine on the weekends and then store them in individual servings in the freezer. I keep a wide variety of frozen entrées in individual servings in my freezer at all times. It is great to have something to *go to* when you are tired or busy and need something flavorful. I must say, my freezer meals keep me out of the fast food joints and away from store-bought frozen dinners, most of which have little flavor and are often loaded with trans fats and sodium.

You're probably thinking that it takes time to do all this cooking and freezing. Well, you are correct. You will need to decide if it is worth it for you to add this approach to your family Routine. Getting the children to help with the cooking on the weekend might be a good way to teach them some life skills while spending quality time together. You can always toss in a recipe for homemade cookies now and then to spice things up.

If you have children and a spouse, you could let everyone have a choice as to what they would like to eat on a busy evening.

There are many times when families eat dinner or lunch on the run. I am thinking about soccer practice, parents' night at school, dance lessons, or dozens of other activities that leave no time to cook. For fun, you might even prepare a *Freezer Menu* for the kids. Put it on a simple white erase board so that it is easy to change. List the options from your freezer and create a new family Tradition of what you do on those busy evenings. Can't you hear your son or daughter saying, "Mom is tonight *freezer night*?"

I have given you just a few examples of foods that I enjoy cooking and eating. They are healthy but not diet food. I use real butter, real sugar, and real whole foods. As you already know, I do not use trans fats or artificial sweeteners. I try to stick to whole grains while limiting white flour and sugar but I am not rigid about this. What I am doing is not perfect, but it is working for me. You will need to find your own *go to* foods and recipes. You might even decide that you aren't into cooking and teach yourself how to eat healthy while mostly eating at restaurants. Again, you must find your own way.

My Habits, Routines, Rituals, and Traditions for my diet are still evolving. I occasionally get tired of cooking and eat out for a while, or have a favorite dish that I eat for lunch every day for a month, or stop making my tortilla soup for a few months. What I eat varies as my schedule, social life, work, and mood changes.

I have shared some of my eating Habits and Routines to help you get started but you must find your own way as you explore your own HRRTs and decide how you want to manage your diet. Believe in yourself! I know you can do it! And don't forget to take it in MicroSteps.

RESOURCES

Below is a list of books, television shows, websites, and social media resources that I have found helpful. The list is not comprehensive, but it includes things that helped me and I hope will help you. My intention is to point out the value of seeking knowledge—because knowledge is the best way to work toward a healthier body and self.

There are numerous books on depression, anxiety, self-esteem, fashion, how to shop, cooking, and nutrition that could be helpful. Hundreds of websites, blogs, twitter accounts, television shows, and organizations offer endless opportunity to learn new things.

Take these suggestions below only if they are interesting to you and then approach them in MicroSteps. Let your brain live a little! There is no test. Enjoy!

BOOKS

Costin, Carolyn, MA, MED, MFT, *The Eating Disorder Sourcebook*, Third Edition, McGraw-Hill Companies, 2007.

Cowen, Dolly, MA, MFT and Goldklang, Lynne, MA, MFT, *Count It as a Vegetable and Move On: Ending the Food-Abuse / Self-Abuse Cycle of the Typical Dieter*, The Nurturing Connection and Isaac, Nathan Pub. Co., Inc., 2001.

Kelly, Clinton and London, Stacy (Hosts of TLC's What not to Wear), *Dress Your Best*, Three Rivers Press, an imprint of Crown Publishing Group, a division of Random House, Inc., New York, 2005.

Kessler, David A., MD, *The End of Overeating. Taking Control of the Insatiable American Appetite*, Rodale Inc., 2009.

London, Stacy, The Truth About Style, Furry Perry, Inc., Viking, The Penguin Group, 2012.

Preston, John D., Psy.D., *Lift Your Mood Now: Simple Things You Can Do to Beat the Blues,* New Harbinger Publications, Inc. (If you cannot locate the book, Google the author. He has a website: www.psyd-fx.com. All his books are wonderful), 2009.

Schiraldi, Glenn R., Ph.D., *The Self-Esteem Workbook,* New Harbinger Publications, Inc., 2001.

Wolf, Anthony E., Ph.D. *Get Out of My Life but First Could You Drive Me and Cheryl to the Mall*, Harper Collins Canada Ltd, (This is a parents' guide to teenagers. It is old but amazing. My sister still thanks me for this suggested reading and her children are now adults.), 1991.

Vigilante, *Kevin,* MD, MPH, and Flynn, Mary, Ph.D., *Low-Fat Lies High-Fat Frauds and the Healthiest Diet in the World* , LifeLine Press, a Regnery Publishing Company, Washington, DC., 2009.

And, of course:

Cookbooks! Cookbooks! Cookbooks! Just pick your favorite. Whether you are just learning to cook or a seasoned chef, cookbooks can provide you with additional resources and ideas.

TELEVISION SHOWS, ORGANIZATIONS, GROUPS, AND PLACES TO INCREASE KNOWLEDGE

The television show *What Not to Wear* used to be on *The Learning Channel*. It can help you in learning to dress the body you have, dressing the body as it changes, and in keeping up with what is fashionable so that you have confidence as you shop; this has a very positive impact on self-esteem. It is still possible to purchase the DVDs on Amazon.

The Food Network and the *Cooking Channel* can be a great help in learning to cook. Some of the shows offer instructions for cooking healthy and others not so much. Regardless of what the show is teaching, it is an opportunity to improve cooking skills and get some ideas.

The *Weight Watchers Organization* can be a support if you need help in learning to eat a healthy balanced diet. This is one way to learn about nutrition. You can participate online or in person.

Your local *HMO (Health Maintenance Organization)* or *hospital* may offer classes in exercise or nutrition. Mine offers yoga, exercising for seniors, general exercise classes, and nutrition classes. All for free as part of my health insurance.

A *college class* is a great place to learn. You don't have to work on a degree to take a class. Even if you already have a college degree or maybe even a graduate degree, you could still audit a class in nutrition or cooking.

Adult school and *local learning centers* are available in most cities and even small towns. Local professionals often offer classes at a low fee or even free as a way of marketing their business. You can benefit from these classes and perhaps increase your social support.

Dance classes, GYMs, Department of Recreation, and *sports teams* are just a few ideas of ways to get off the sofa and into the action. As you know, I am not into the GYM but that does not mean you won't like it.

WEBSITES

www.nutritiondata.com Self Nutrition Data is a place to get nutrition data about what you are eating.

http://www.cdc.gov/nutrition/everyone/basics/carbs.html Center for Disease Control and Prevention offers Basic Nutrition Information.

http://caloriecount.about.com/ Calorie Count helps with counting calories on over 250,000 different foods.

http://www.eatright.org/ Academy of Nutrition and Dietetics is a great resource for all types of information related for food and diet.

http://www.carolyncostin.com/about.php Carolyn Costin is an internationally recognized expert on Eating Disorders with residential facilities in California, Oregon, and New York.

http://www.obesity.org/ The Obesity Society's mission statement says, "Through research, education, and advocacy, to better understand, prevent, and treat obesity and improve the lives of those affected." Their website has a lot of great information and resources.

http://www.hindawi.com/journals/jobe/ Journal of Obesity states on their website that they are "a peer-reviewed, open access journal that publishes original research articles, review articles, and clinical studies in all areas of obesity." They offer a lot of good information.

These four websites offer a lot of great recipes and meal ideas. The recipes are not all healthy but many are.

http://allrecipes.com/Default.aspx

http://www.tasteofhome.com/

http://www.foodnetwork.com/

https://www.kashi.com/

BLOGS, TWITTER, AND FACEBOOK

There is so much information online that I chose not to make a list because the sites open, close, and change frequently. Instead, I want you to explore Twitter, Blogs, and Facebook Accounts as they interest you. Each is a great place to join a conversation, gain information, or find support.

The following list of words would be a good starting place when you sit down to do a Google or Yahoo search: nutrition, obesity, parenting, depression, anxiety, weight management, exercise, and fitness. The truth is that you can put any word that is on your mind into the search engine and come up with endless resources.

Check out me on Twitter at *@SueSpeakeLMFT*. Learn how Twitter works. It is a great place to track down information. By the time you read this, I will have a website, a blog, and hope to continue to offer you support in your journey to a healthy, average size body.

ACKNOWLEDGMENTS

This book would be but a pile of scribbled notes on my desk had it not been for Sylvia Cary, LMFT, my friend, editor, and author of numerous books including *The Therapist Writer*. In addition to editing, she taught me how to take my pile of notes and turn them into a book. I had no idea how challenging a task that would be but she stuck with me throughout the process.

I can honestly say that my life would not be the same without Sandie Einbinder. We met when she was a social worker in the Department of Adult Protective services and I was her daughter's Kindergarten teacher. She has been a support, a friend, a mother, and a kick me in the butt when I need it person in my life for over thirty years.

My dear friend, psychologist Susan Harper Slate, has been a support, inspiration, and an insightful challenger over the years. The self-confidence I gained in the course of our friendship gave me the courage to tell my story. Thank you also to her husband, attorney Daniel Slate, for his encouragement and support.

I am so grateful to Audrey Newman and Ray Wilson for their love and support at a time in my life when I needed it. Thank you for the wisdom and guidance shared.

I would like to thank my family, especially my sister Marcella and her children, for their unconditional support when I was so busy with work and writing that I had no time to spend with them. They are always there.

Thank you to my friend Ceri Hulugalle for her support and to the Writers of Kern for sharing their talents and time. I especially want to thank Dennis VanderWerff, Dana Martin, Annis Cassels, Terry Redman, and Joan Raymond for their special support.

A special thank you goes to Rhoda Lurie from RhoDesigns for her generosity and fashion guidance. Thank you to Dotti Albertine for her time and support. Thank you to Judy Alfter for her support.

Then there are those amazingly generous people who took the time from their busy lives to read various chapters and drafts of the book. Your support, suggestions, and critiques made all the difference. Your feedback gave me the confidence and courage to continue writing.

Finally, to my cats Oliver and Poppy who always seem to know when to jump up onto the keyboard and disrupt my focus.

ABOUT THE AUTHOR

SUE SPEAKE grew up in Texas and moved to California in her twenties. She taught elementary school for seventeen years. While teaching elementary school, she went back college at California State University at Northridge to earn a Master's Degree. Sue is a Licensed Marriage and Family Therapist who has been serving patients in Southern and Central California for over twenty years. Her experience as a therapist covers all ages and many issues, including substance abuse. She has worked with groups, families, couples, and individuals providing support for chronic and severe issues as well as offering a little support to help folks get through a difficult time.

Sue received a Bachelor of Science Degree in Education, with an Early Childhood Specialization from North Texas State University (aka University of Texas) in 1975. She received an Elementary Teacher's Certificate in Texas that same year. Sue earned a Master's of Science Degree in Marriage, Family, and Child Counseling from California State University Northridge in 1991 and became a California Licensed Marriage and Family Therapist in 1994. Sue became a California Licensed Professional Clinical Counselor in 2013.

While writing, working with patients, hanging out with friends and family take up much of her time, Sue also enjoys growing herbs, roses, cooking, and learning just about anything. Spending time with her two cats, Oliver and Poppy, is a favorite way to relax with a good book or a favorite show.

MicroSteps®

Dear Reader,

MicroSteps® Therapy (MST) has applications beyond weight management. When someone is stuck, unable to move forward, MST is a clinical tool that may be helpful. I look forward to sharing more about this with you in the days to come.

Warmly,
Sue

www.ingramcontent.com/pod-product-compliance
Lightning Source LLC
Chambersburg PA
CBHW031502270326
41930CB00006B/203